A HISTORY OF DENTISTRY IN CANADA

D. W. GULLETT

A history of dentistry
in Canada

PUBLISHED FOR
THE CANADIAN DENTAL ASSOCIATION BY
UNIVERSITY OF TORONTO PRESS

© University of Toronto Press 1971
Printed in Canada
by University of Toronto Press
Toronto and Buffalo
ISBN 0-8020-1759-2
Microfiche ISBN 0-8020-0048-7
LC 79-151370

Our professional ancestors
have passed on to us standards
of value based on accumulative experience,
and these standards have become a part
of the spirit of dentistry.
Therefore, it is important that
we rescue some of the ideals of the past
and use them in charting the
course for the future.

P. G. Anderson
Associate Dean
Faculty of Dentistry
University of Toronto
1955

Contents

Preface

The development of the art and science of dentistry in Canada parallels the historical development of the country as a whole with considerable exactitude. At the time of Confederation in 1867, dentistry had developed as a recognizable profession. As further provinces became identified one by one with Confederation, so too were their dental professions ready for identification. Few like to admit that time of war is one of progress. Yet three wars – the Boer War and the two world wars – in which Canada as a nation has been a participant, mark significant periods of advancement in Canadian dentistry.

Archaeological records show that man has suffered from dental diseases from early times. Through the ages dentistry in various forms has been practised by many types of practitioners. It was on the North American continent, however, and during the first half of the nineteenth century, that dentistry first became a separate profession. The formation of the Society of Surgeon Dentists of the City and State of New York in 1834 and of the American Society of Dental Surgeons in 1840, the establishment of the *American Journal of Dental Science* in 1839, and the chartering of the Baltimore College of Dental Surgery in 1840 set a pattern for dentistry not to be found elsewhere in the world. The development of the dental profession in Canada and the United States has been along parallel lines.

It has been well said that a country which is not interested in its past either has none or is ashamed of it. This is equally true of a profession within a country. It is impossible to comprehend the present, much less guess at the future, without knowledge of the past. The present is so close to us, of so immediate and pressing importance, that we are inclined to forget that our predecessors had problems, so different from and yet comparable to ours.

History, to be worthy of the name, must be not only descriptive of that of which we are proud, but also not guilty of excluding that which we may not regard with pride. The dental profession constitutes but a small section of society and for an understanding of its attitudes and actions it is necessary to know something of the environs of society as a whole.

To one who chose to become a dentist during his seventh year, and has never regretted the choice, the gathering together of the facts related herein has been a labour of love. The selection from voluminous subject matter and the writing of the text has been difficult and laborious. Every statement of fact has been reasonably documented. For the comments upon the factual information I accept responsibility. In several instances information handed down over the years was found at variance with original sources. Special care has been exercised respecting such instances.

The plan of the book was established to cover the development of Canadian dentistry, but with room for detailed accounts of the history of the profession in individual provinces. Organizations within the profession have altered titles from time to time: the policy has been to use the title current at the time of reference. My original ambition was to include all significant achievements with due credit to the dentists responsible. In order to keep within reasonable bounds, however, it became necessary to be selective and concise.

I have had the full co-operation of the various dental organizations, dental libraries, and other professional bodies in compiling basic information. A great number of individual dentists have assisted in establishing facts and it is not possible to list them all here. A few, who have exceeded what might be expected of any individual, are: G.M. Dewis of Halifax, C.C. Bourne and Mervyn A. Rogers of Montreal, Conrad Godin of Three Rivers, John Clay of Calgary, and J.D. Hawkins of Edmonton. The late Paul-E. Poitras of Montreal left a large private collection of historical items on dentistry, which I have had the pleasure of studying. J. Stanley Bagnall of Halifax, during his latter years, compiled voluminous historical notes from the literature which I have utilized.

Much information has come from archives and reference libraries, and credit appears in the text for the main items from these sources. However, I should like to express my gratitude for the courteous and generous assistance given during my visits and for the care exercised in replying to my numerous letters of inquiry to: British Columbia Provincial Archives, Victoria; Glenbow Foundation, Calgary; Saskatchewan Provincial Archives, Regina; Manitoba Provincial Archives, Winnipeg; Royal Ontario Museum, Toronto; Toronto Reference Library; Ontario Archives, Toronto; Montreal City Library – Gagnon Collection; Archives du Québec, Quebec; New Brunswick Museum, Saint John; The Public Archives, Halifax; Public Archives of Canada, Ottawa. I am greatly indebted to Dr W.G. McIntosh, who read the manuscript and made valuable suggestions and to Mr Ian Montagnes of University of Toronto Press for his sage advice and counsel.

Without the patience and assistance of my wife, Alice, this book would not have been possible. She has done practically all the typing and assisted at each stage of preparation.

D.W.G.

Willowdale, Ontario

A HISTORY OF DENTISTRY IN CANADA

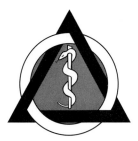

Official emblem of dentistry in Canada

1
The first Canadians

The development of a profession is inextricably related to the history of the country wherein it exists. Advanced professions are not formed in underdeveloped countries. (This is not to say, however, that in developed countries all professions need be equally advanced. Some may lag.) The history of Canada is a short one, but during it the dental profession has advanced rapidly and progressively along with its homeland. The advance has not been even from coast to coast. Canada is the second largest country in the world, exceeded in area only by the USSR. Its development has occurred by regions, which gradually were united in a federation of provinces. In much the same way the segments of society, including the professions, have grown regionally and been co-ordinated.

Geography has always played an important part in the history of Canada. The pattern of settlement was along the southern border in clusters which eventually coalesced into a ribbon of population stretching 4,000 miles from the Atlantic to the Pacific. As population increased, the ribbon widened northward. Because of the size of Canada and the distribution of its people, organization in all phases often proved difficult. It is easily understood that individuals living on the Atlantic side might think quite differently from those on the Pacific side, particularly when comparatively few Canadians ever travel completely across their own country. These facts are basic to an understanding of the nature and progress of a profession from birth to maturity.

Toothache and other dental disorders arrived in Canada, insofar as we can guess, with the first inhabitants. Our knowledge of conditions among the early Indians and Eskimos is recent and fragmentary, based on the research of anthropologists, but the evidence suggests that the incidence of dental disease was high indeed before the white man came to this continent.

Among some Indian cultures, ossuary burials occurred approximately every ten years. At such times a 'Feast of the Dead' was held, and the village dead were exhumed from their individual primary graves and reburied in a common large pit. A considerable number of these ossuary sites are known and two of them near Toronto (the Robb and Fairty sites) have been carefully excavated during recent years. Both have been dated to the 1500s. An analysis of finds at the Fairty site, involving a study of approximately 36,000 bones with the expected proportion of upper and lower jaws, has been published.[1] It states:

Premortem loss of teeth has occurred in 44% of maxillae and in 77% of mandibles. The ages represented are: prepubertal – 28%; adolescent – 14%; adults – 58%. About 20% of jaws are with periodontal disease and abscess formation. Molars have the highest evidence of premortem loss, followed by premolars and canines.

The incidence of caries in remaining teeth was: lower molars, 62%; upper molars, 53%; premolars, 13%; canines, 7%; incisors, 6%. The incidence of hypercementosis was: upper molars, 47%; lower molars, 35%; canines, 20%; incisors, 7%. At the pre-Iroquois Robb site, caries were found in abundance, along with periodontal disease and considerable cementosis.[2] Much the same incidence of dental disease was discovered at a Huron ossuary site near Midland, Ontario, dated to 1636: the burial ceremony is described by Father Brébeuf in the Jesuit Relations.[3] One further example, a pre-Iroquois burial in Ontario known as the Bosomworth Site, contained the bones of at least 15 adults and nine children.[4] All adult skulls showed signs of dental pathology: caries, attrition, premortem tooth loss, and alveolar abscesses were common, as well as slight evidence of periodontal disease.

On the basis of such evidence, Indians must have suffered severe pain from dental disease. We can only guess how they treated it: their medicine men belonged to a secret society and little is known of their practices. However, the discovery of jawbones with one or more teeth, or indeed all of them, removed before death suggests that some manner of extraction had occurred. In some cases it appears that heroic action was taken, resulting in the removal not only of the tooth but of the alveolar process.

In others the tooth appears to have been removed without destruction of surrounding tissues.

Writings on the medicine man are confined largely to descriptions of an Indian, elaborately dressed in skins and feathers, who performed complicated magical ceremonies. It is known, however, that a second type of medicine man existed, who dressed in ordinary fashion and treated the sick with various herbs. A compendium of Indian medicinal plants and their applications has been established.[5] It lists poultices made from the leaves, bark or roots of several different kinds of wild plants, and it is reasonable to assume that these were used to treat abscessed teeth. Specific herbal remedies are given for toothache: 'Iris-root inserted in a cavity will kill nerve, tooth will come out'; 'bit of [yarrow] root inserted in hollow tooth for toothache.' In desert regions of North America, turtle back was commonly referred to as 'toothache plant,' and the dried leaves were chewed on the side of the mouth that hurt. There are even suggestions of preventive dentistry. In his exhaustive study, *The Bella Coola Indians*, T.F. McIlwraith noted: 'When a milk tooth is lost, anyone who happens to be present, should pick it up, pass it four times around the child's head sunwise and throw it away.' No explanation for this West Coast custom is given, but in this respect Indian folklore was no more mysterious (or unfounded) than some followed today.

There is reason to believe that the incidence of dental disease varied considerably among the Indians. An English surgeon wrote in 1885 that he had seen Indian skulls with perfect dentitions at York Factory, where he was employed by the Hudson's Bay Company.[6] In some cases the teeth were well worn down, which he attributed to the habit of chewing pitch. On the other hand, he stated that Indians suffered a great deal from toothache, and that aphous and ulcerative stomatitis epidemics were annual occurrences. Considerable variation in the incidence of caries was reported from area to area among modern Crees and Chipewayans in a study published in 1930.[7] The Indians examined were for the most part adults, and the numbers involved were small. At Fitzgerald and Fort Smith, 54% of the men had sound teeth, but at Fond-du-lac the incidence of sound teeth skyrocketed to 76% for the women and 94% for the men. The author commented: 'If to have sound teeth be the mark of a pure Indian, and if to have carious teeth an indication that there is a strain of white blood in the stock, then the Fond-du-lac men and women are the purest.'

Behind this statement seems to be the belief, held for many years, that the white man brought dental disease to the native peoples of North America. Anthropological evidence does not support this theory. Some exceptional finds have been made, it is true. One of the most exciting archaeological discoveries in eastern North America, made at Port au Choix, Newfoundland, in the summer of 1968, revealed skeletal remains that by radiocarbon test are 4,300 years old. Virtually no dental caries could be found in them, though many individuals had very worn teeth with the pulp cavity often exposed, resulting in apical abscesses.[8] This evidence indicates that dental caries did not in fact exist among Indians at that early date, at least not in this tribe. On the other hand, a study of an Ohio Indian burial ground, dated to 900 AD, revealed that 70% of the people had abscessed teeth, more than half had lost one or more teeth from periodontal disease, and only three out of 103 skulls did not show tooth decay.[9] The difference, if any, before and after the white man's arrival appears to be one of percentage in the incidence of dental disease rather than its absence or presence.

Across Canada there were some fifty different Indian tribes. Among them the prevalence of dental disease varied considerably. Generally, this variation has been attributed to diet. It is said that corn planters such as the Iroquois were prone to tooth decay because of their mush diet, whereas those hunters whose diet was almost exclusively of protein and fat were almost immune to caries. Methods of treatment for dental disorder varied as well from tribe to tribe. The herbs employed were those near at hand. The Iroquois used blue flag for toothache. The Ojibway used camas root. The Haida cauterized the nerve of a decayed tooth with a sharp sliver of flint, and chewed spruce gum to keep their teeth white. The Beothuks of Newfoundland gave teething infants inflated fish bladders to chew on. To categorize dental diseases and treatments among the Indian tribes would be an interesting but most difficult task.

The Eskimo is noted for the use he makes of the few natural resource materials available to him in the Arctic. His carvings in stone, ivory and bone in particular have gained for him a high reputation. The ingenuity of one Eskimo is shown in the accompanying illustration. During his travels on the fringes of the white man's civilization this man found a vulcanite denture with central and lateral incisor teeth. It so happened that the same teeth were missing in his own mouth, together with some others. From ivory he proceeded to carve teeth to fit the extra spaces in his mouth, bored holes in the vulcanite, and tied the pieces of ivory in proper position. He wore the denture, we are told, with a considerable degree of pride. Now it is in the museum of the Faculty of Dentistry, University of Toronto.

In 1939, C.H.M. Williams of that faculty investigated dental health among Eskimos of Canada's Eastern Arctic.[10] Among his findings were: that immunity to caries existed, except among those Eskimo with access to white man's food; that susceptibility to periodontitis was almost universal; that the roots of Eskimo teeth are surprisingly short and sharply tapered; and that considerable mobility of teeth existed by age 45, with 20% of teeth per individual missing.

The Eskimos had their shamans, corresponding in many respects to the medicine men of the Indians. Some were trained by apprenticeship, while others received their powers through a sudden vision. They used juggling tricks, but their usual practice was to induce in themselves a kind of temporary dementia and in that condition give utterance to more or less incoherent ravings, which the laity interpreted as instruction from oracles which would drive out the evil spirits. Eskimos were ignorant of herbal medicines but could bandage a wound and were capable of using splints for a broken limb.[11]

The first dentist to visit the Canadian Arctic was W.P. Millar of Edmonton, who went in response to the urging of the Hudson's Bay Com-

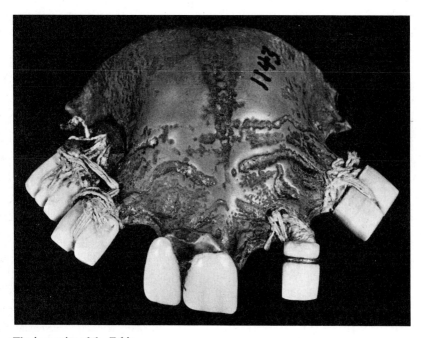

The ingenuity of the Eskimo

pany post managers in the far north. Millar spent six months during the summer of 1922 travelling some eight thousand miles, down the Mackenzie River, then west, and back via Bering Strait to Vancouver. At every landing along the way he was met by dental sufferers who were ready to fight for a place in his operating chair. According to the published account of the trip, the Eskimos were very receptive to the services offered but the Indians were suspicious. Along the way, Millar employed as an assistant an Eskimo named Mike, who at the end of the journey asked if he could buy the equipment. Millar jokingly named a price. To his surprise, 'Mike pulled out a roll of Canadian currency sufficient to choke an ox and immediately became the possessor of the apparatus.' Mike loaded the equipment on his sleigh, and drove his team of huskies into the unknown eastern Arctic.[12] Until his death in 1930, he wandered across the Arctic region extracting teeth, becoming a small legend as 'Siberian Mike,' the Eskimo's dentist. Presumably, the task was not difficult, owing to his patients' susceptibility to periodontitis and the short tapered roots of their teeth.

Practically all accounts of early Canadian history relate, with considerable variation, how Jacques Cartier and his men suffered from scurvy during the winter of 1535–6, while they were frozen in near the site of the present city of Quebec. Cartier himself wrote a narrative of the voyage, which was published as a small book (*Bref récit*) in 1545. Of the 110 Frenchmen, the disease eventually killed 25 and all but three were disabled. In despair, an autopsy was performed on the body of one of the first victims, Philippe Rougemont of Amboise. This was the first postmortem in Canadian history, but unfortunately, it gave no clue to a remedy. Cartier's book is of particular interest to dentists, because of its description of the oral manifestations of the disease: 'And all the sick had their mouths so tainted and their gums so decayed that the flesh peeled off down to the roots of their teeth while the latter all fell out in turn.' All would have probably perished miserably, had not the captain noticed that an Indian named Dom Agaya, who two weeks earlier had been suffering from the disease, had regained his strength and health. Through careful inquiry, it was discovered that the Indian remedy was to boil the bark and sap of a tree, 'then to drink of the same decoction every other day and to put the dregges of it upon the legges that is sick'.[13] The Indians termed the tree *annedda* or 'Tree of Life'; various investigators have referred to it as white cedar, spruce, or other evergreen. Within eight days the men were well. The account constitutes the first recorded description of a disease on this continent and, from the standpoint of dentistry, the first record of oral disease.

Folklore has come down through the years that Champlain brought a dentist with him on his expedition to the new world during the early seventeenth century. This could not be true, because dentists as such did not exist at that time. However, Louis Hébert, an apothecary, did accompany Champlain, first to the ill-fated Acadian settlement on the Bay of Fundy and then, after returning to France, to Quebec. The designation of apothecary had a wider meaning then than today. The apothecary practised medicine, and undoubtedly Hébert would have extracted teeth and performed emergency dental treatment in both new colonies. The names of several barber-surgeons who also accompanied Champlain on his trips and stayed at Quebec on a more or less temporary basis are recorded, but Hébert has a special place in history as the first real Canadian settler, having brought his wife and family and erected the first house in Quebec. He served as the first practitioner of health services in Canada until his death in 1627 from a fall on the ice.[14]

The first physician in New France was Robert Giffard, a French naval surgeon, who came out on a trading venture in 1627. In 1634 he was granted the seigneury of Beauport, where he built a home and entered into the first private colonizing enterprise by bringing out settlers and their families. In 1640 he became the first doctor of the Hôtel-Dieu, Quebec, the first hospital in the colony. Giffard continued his activities, engaging in colonization and fur-trading, as well as medical practice. He died at Beauport in 1668.[15]

Beginning in the thirteenth century, guilds of barber-surgeons were formed in Europe, probably first in France and then in England, Germany and some other countries. Originally, the barbers owed their business largely to the fact that after the monks were forbidden by the Pope to wear beards, smooth chins and shaving became a general fashion. Physicians of the era considered the letting of blood was necessary but beneath their dignity, and were glad to relegate the task to the barbers. Gradually, the activities of the latter came to include bleeding, cupping, leeching, the giving of enemas, and the extracting of teeth. The guilds of barber-surgeons became established by royal decrees, limiting the services that could be performed and establishing examinations by appointed senior members for admission to the guild. Eventually, the surgeons separated from the barbers and formed guilds of their own. This separation took place in England in 1745, and at a later date in France.[16]

Jean Madry, the first barber-surgeon in Quebec, arrived about 1651 and eventually succeeded Giffard in charge of Hôtel Dieu. In 1663 he was appointed by Royal Commission of Louis XIV lieutenant in New France of the chief barber-surgeon of the King, and authorized to establish 'the mastership of a school of barber-surgeons in the locality, so that the town of Quebec and also all places, towns, villages and settlements under obedience to the King, all those passing through or sojourning there may be well and safely treated ...'[17] As a barber-surgeon, Madry was qualified to extract teeth.

The first directory in Canada was published in 1791, and listed those practising the healing arts.[18] At this period, Lower Canada (later Quebec) had a population of approximately 110,000 (100,000 French- and 10,000 English-speaking) and Upper Canada (later Ontario) fewer than 20,000. The practitioners listed were located only in the larger centres, Quebec and Montreal, where examining boards for licences existed. The manner of listing suggests that the age of specialization was already in existence at this early date. Nineteen practitioners appear in Quebec and 33 in Montreal. For Montreal, the names are grouped under the categories for which they were licensed to practise – physicians, surgeons, accouchers, apothecaries, and *saigneurs et aracheurs de dents* (blood-letters and tooth-drawers). Of the last category, there were nine. While these men engaged in little dentistry beyond extraction, they must be considered the forerunners of the dental profession in Canada. The great-grandson of one of them, Stephen Globensky, became one of the most prominent dentists in Montreal 75 years later. With the exception of seven or possibly eight, the names listed are French, and for the most part they were most likely trained in France. Probably it would be wrong to think of these men as practising their profession exclusively, because for many years to come it would still be necessary to have some additional occupation in order to make a living. This was partly due to the economy of the colony and also to lack of appreciation of the health sciences. It is said that the father of surgery, Ambrose Paré, a couple of centuries earlier made his living in France by cutting hair and shaving in order to work as a surgeon.

By the end of the eighteenth century, the type of practice carried out by the barber-surgeons was rapidly dying. As in other branches of the healing arts, a new kind of dentistry was developing, influenced greatly in Canada by the developments which occurred in the United States.

2
Early colonial period
1800-1839

Pierre Fauchard (1678–1761) of Paris is justly recognized as the father of modern dentistry. One of the founders of the dental profession in the United States, Chapin A. Harris, has said of him, 'He found dental art a crude branch of mechanics; he left it a digested and systematic branch of the curative art.' No single individual in the entire history of dentistry exerted a stronger influence upon its development. His book, *Le chirurgien dentist*, is the most famous of all books in the field and made him the pioneer of modern dental thought. He was the first of a group of renowned dentists of France who followed rapidly during the eighteenth century. Whether or not he coined the title 'Surgeon Dentist' is not clear, but he became known for this in any event.

The level of dental skill in his lifetime is indicated by discoveries made in 1966 during the restoration of the Fortress of Louisburg, Cape Breton Island. Two of the men buried in the King's Chapel of the fortress had metallic fillings in their teeth. The material of the fillings was investigated with an electron probe microanalyzer.[1] One filling was found in one burial: a mesial cavity in the first upper left molar was partially filled with lead, apparently in the form of a thin foil. In the other burial, fillings were present in both lower first molars, and in each case, the metal used was tin. The latter skeleton has been identified as that of the Duc d'Anville, who died in 1746 and was reburied beneath the chapel in 1749. These skulls represent one of the earliest examples, if not the earliest, of dental restoration found within the boundaries of what became Canada. Undoubtedly, the fillings were inserted in France.

During the American Revolution rapport between France and the

United States was high, and many French troops crossed the Atlantic to join the battle against the British. Among them were dentists, disciples of Fauchard, a number of whom remained in America. Their influence was great: established precedents did not exist in the New World, and new ideas were quickly absorbed. They were not wholly responsible for the development of the profession in the United States (before the Revolution, a few dentists had already come from England and France to practise in Boston and other cities), but the influence of these French dentists of the 1770s was the single most important factor during the period, extending beyond their direct work. The New World thus gained the legacy of dental knowledge of Fauchard, Le Farge, Bourdet and Bunon of France, together with that of John Hunter, Thomas Berdmore, William Green, and John Watts of England. The new arrivals broke through the barriers of secrecy which surrounded dental practice in their countries of origin. Though comparatively few, they acted as preceptors – pioneers of dental education. In a comparatively short time, the number of native dentists increased through the apprenticeship training they offered.

Shortly after the turn of the century, dentists who had some degree of apprenticeship training began to come to Canada from the United States. For the most part, these men visited the larger centres of population, Montreal, Quebec, and York (later Toronto); gradually, some of them established practice on a more or less permanent basis. At that time, Canada still consisted of only two provinces, Lower and Upper Canada, the former with 250,000 inhabitants, the latter with 70,000. Nova Scotia, New Brunswick, Prince Edward Island, and Newfoundland were separate colonies to which dentists from the United States also came. The main trade route of the period between Canada and the United States ran from Montreal via Lake Champlain to New York and Boston. It was natural that dentists arrived first by this path.

Contemporary information respecting these early practitioners is to be found, for the most part, in their newspaper advertisements. The first such announcement found in Nova Scotia appeared in the *Acadian Recorder* of 3 December 1814:

Mr. Hume, Surgeon, has removed into New House in Barrington Street, 2 doors south of the Baptist Meeting House, He will also operate as a Dentist in fixing Artificial Teeth etc. etc.

The origins of Hume have not been established, but from the advertisement it can be assumed that he was a surgeon who had picked up some knowledge of dentistry. This was a common circumstance for many years.

Probably the assumption may also be made that he came from England. A survey of early advertisements establishes that a few of these practitioners came directly to Canada from England, although the general flow was from the south.

It is of interest to know something of the degree of proficiency which had been reached in dentistry. The length of training that Canada's early practitioners received would have varied greatly, as the only form of agreement was indentureship contract between preceptor and pupil, not always fulfilled. Josiah Flagg was one of the outstanding dentists of the time. In 1796 he published the following advertisement in a Boston newspaper, which in 1875 was reproduced in the *Boston Medical Journal*.

Josiah Flagg, surgeon dentist – informs the public that he practises in all the branches with improvements, i.e. transplants both live and dead teeth with just conveniency, and gives less pain than that heretofore practised in Europe or America; extracts teeth and stumps or roots with ease; reinstates teeth and gums that are much depreciated by nature, carelessness, acids, or wasted at the roots; regulates teeth from their first cutting to prevent fever and pain in children, assists nature in the extension of the jaws for the beautiful arrangement of the second set and preserves them in their natural whiteness. Entirely free from all scorbutis complaints. And when thus put in order and his directions followed (which are simple), he engages that the further care of a dentist will be wholly unnecessary; eases pain in teeth without drawing, stops bleeding in the gums, jaws or arteries; lines and plumbs teeth with virgin gold, foil or lead. Fixes gold roofs and palates, and artificial teeth of any quality without injury to, and independent of the natural ones; greatly assisting the pronunciation and the swallow, when injured by natural or other defects. A room for the practice, with every accommodation at his house, where may be had dentifrices, tinctures, teeth and gum brushes, mastice etc. warranted, approved and adapted to the various ages and circumstances; also charr-sticks particularly useful in cleaning the fore teeth and preserving a natural whiteness; which medicine and charr-sticks are to be sold wholesale and retail that they may be more extensively useful. Dr. Flagg has a method to furnish those ladies and gentlemen or children with artificial teeth, gold, gums, roots or palates, that are at a distance and cannot attend him personally.

Cash given for handsome and healthy live teeth at No. 47 Newburg Street, Boston, 1796.

Among the early dentists to come from Vermont was Levi Spear Parmly, who practised at Montreal for a short time and then continued at Quebec

THE

SUMMUM
BONUM.

BY

LEVI S. PARMLY,

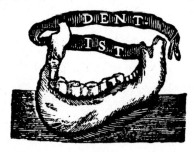

AND

Medical Electrician;

━━━━━➔➘⦂⦂◦⦂⦂◀◀━━━━━

No. 2, Palace Street, Quebec,

August 29th, A. D. 1815.

Title page of the first book on dentistry
published in Canada

PR NTED BY J. NEILSON, MOUNTAIN STREET

City. While in Quebec, he published in 1815 the first Canadian book on
dentistry, a work of 65 pages entitled *Summum Bonum*. An original copy
of the book is in the Gagnon Collection of the Montreal City Library, and
the type of practice can be determined from the fee schedule it contains.

Any advice given gratis.
Prices for the following are as circumstances present themselves.
A full set of teeth with gold springs not to exceed one hundred dollars.
A single tooth not to exceed ten dollars.
Evening the teeth not to exceed one dollar.
Separating the teeth not to exceed one dollar.
For mending a tooth with foil one dollar, gold etc.

Teeth made white and polished, price depends on the state and number of the teeth; from one to five dollars – not the least pain under the operation.
Tooth paste etc. etc. for keeping the breath, teeth and gums agreeable.
Deranged and ulcer teeth extracted gratis, with as great care and ease as any operator.
My first wish is a continuance of the public's patronage – my highest ambition to deserve it.

The Quebec Almanac for the year 1816 still listed five *saigneurs et aracheurs de dents* (barber surgeons), but this type of practitioner was being replaced by dentists, many of them itinerants. Among such men was Eleazer Gidney, one of the most successful and prominent dentists of his generation. After completing three years of apprenticeship, Gidney gained a licence to practise physic and surgery in New York State. He practised for a brief period, but by the autumn of 1817 was studying dentistry at Baltimore and New York. He practised dentistry for a short time at Utica, NY, and then came to York (Toronto), where he practised during 1825. In February 1826 he left York and went to Quebec City, bearing a letter of introduction from Christopher Widmer, president of the Medical Board of York, to James Forbes, Deputy Inspector of Hospitals, Quebec. The letter read:

I certify that Eleazer Gidney has resided in this village during the year past and pursued the business of a dentist. I take great pleasure in certifying that he sustains a fair and irreproachable character; and from a knowledge and some experience, I feel authorized to state that he is a man of skill and judgement in his profession.

Gidney stayed in Quebec City for a few months and then left for England where he practised at Manchester. From this time forward he practised for the most part at Manchester, but returned at intervals to practise at New York City and at the end of 1832 returned to York, where his patients included Lady Colborne, wife of the Lieutenant-Governor, and several of her friends. Gidney was one of the most astute men of his time. Wherever he was, his practice consisted of the 'finest people.' He accumulated wealth rapidly by what were for his day the most up-to-date methods.[2]

   These itinerant dentists transported with them a fitted chest of hand instruments. For the most part, these chests were elaborately made of fine

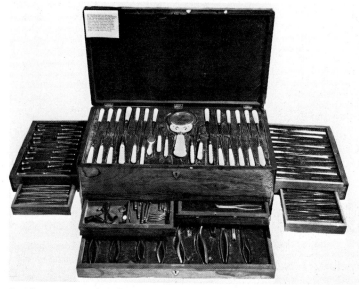

An itinerant's chest of instruments from the mid-nineteenth century

wood, bound with brass, and lined on the inside with velvet. They were fitted with a surprising number of hand instruments (121 in the example illustrated), the handles of which were usually made of ivory, wood, or bone. The instruments were generally manufactured by the dentist himself and exhibit a high degree of technical ability. Quite likely the design of the chest and the large number of instruments were to some measure for the purpose of impressing the patient. Usually visits were advertised in the local newspaper. Some of the itinerants stayed in a place a few days, others a couple of weeks, but seldom for a longer period.

Itinerant dentists continued to visit the larger centres for several decades. One, John Plimpton, who visited Toronto during the 1830s, made his way as far as Prince Edward Island, Newfoundland, and the other Atlantic provinces. To gain some idea of what this entailed, it is necessary to know something of travel conditions of the time. In winter the itinerant dentist journeyed by sleigh, in summer, at first by wagon-like conveyance and later by stage coach over roads hardly entitled to the name. Transportation by water was preferable, when available. By 1840, stagecoaches were running from Toronto to Montreal in the record time of 4½ to 5 days. Canada's first railway, the Champlain and St Lawrence, began operating in 1836, but the first train from Montreal to Toronto did not run until October 1856. Yet under these conditions, the itinerants, with their heavy chests of instruments, travelled long distances.

The ability of these adventurers should not be discounted. In 1913, a Nova Scotian dentist named Daman related how John Plimpton, as an old man, had made a partial denture for his father.[3] Daman was a boy at the time and watched Plimpton hammer out the base plate from an English silver coin and solder on the clasps. The father, he said, wore this denture satisfactorily for many years. Men like Plimpton had ability, and the talent of using available materials for the task at hand.

Resident dentists, or those who set up practice at least on a more or less permanent basis, first appeared in Montreal, the largest population centre. Among these was John Roach Spooner, who arrived during the later 1820s from Vermont, and practised in Montreal until 1841. He gained fame through his discovery of the use of sulphide of arsenic for pulp devitalization. His younger brother, Shearjashub, who apprenticed with him in Montreal and then returned to the United States, published a book on dentistry in 1836 in which he described the use of arsenic, stating that his brother had employed it for several years. Both Spooners were scholarly men. John Spooner never claimed originality for the idea but said frankly that he had discovered it from reading Arabian medical manuscripts, where he had learned that the use of red sulphide of arsenic for relief of pain in teeth was well known by Arabian physicians a thousand years previously. Arsenic was rapidly adopted by other dentists to assist in the removal of the live pulp. Up to this time, two other methods of devitalization had been used: the nerve was cauterized by hot iron, or a sliver of hickory was shaped, carefully slipped in the aperture beside the pulp and given a sharp tap with a mallet. If properly performed, the 'hickory peg' method was *said* to be painless. Arsenic continued to be used in practice until displaced by local anaesthetics more than three-quarters of a century later.

At York, the advertisement of S. Wood, Surgeon Dentist, appeared first in the 4 December 1832 issue of the *Colonial Advocate* and continued to appear in newspapers and directories until 1851. Many names of other practitioners appeared, for periods of varying lengths, in the advertisements of early Toronto newspapers, but Wood's showed remarkable continuity. He was away only one year, 1837, which he spent in New York, Philadelphia, and Boston. On his return his advertisements emphasized that, through his travels, he was in possession of the latest methods of practice, including the use of 'Incorruptible Enamel Teeth' and 'Royal Mineral Cement which, in certain cases, is preferable to any other substance.'[4]

This is the first reference found to the use by a Canadian dentist of what came to be known as amalgam. A Parisian dentist had announced the discovery of a 'silver paste' in 1826, which led to experimentation with several substances in combination with mercury as filling materials. The Crawcour brothers arrived in New York from Paris in 1834, introducing what they called 'Royal Mineral Succedanum.' They promoted this substance with extravagant claims, much to the disgust of the gold foil operators, and bringing about the amalgam war. The controversy caused the destruction of the American Society of Dental Surgeons, the first national dental society. That society passed a resolution declaring it to be malpractice to fill a tooth with amalgam and later expelled any member who refused to pledge himself not to use the material. Apparently, Wood found himself in the midst of the excitement and brought the new material back to Canada.

Little is known about S.C. Parsons, surgeon-dentist of York, except that he published a book of 38 pages in 1830 entitled, *An Essay on the Disorders and Treatment of the Teeth.*[5] At least one original copy of this book exists, in the archives of the University of Maryland (Baltimore College of Dental Surgery). In his introduction, Parsons stated that he had thoroughly investigated the practice of the principal dentists in America, France, and England. Two short extracts from the book give some idea of dental practice in 1830:

OF STOPPING TEETH

Should it be found that the tooth is too far decayed to bear the degree of force which is necessary for applying the gold, pure tin, well prepared, may be used in its stead.

ARTIFICIAL TEETH

The chief object of attention in artificial teeth is, that the substance be durable and not liable to change colour. Human teeth and those of small animals therefore, answers the purpose best, as their enamel is far superior, both in colour and texture to any art can produce. Teeth formed from those of the sea-horse are next in general use, and lately also, they have been formed with great success of fine baked clay, covered with a coat of enamel, after the manner of china, which gives them the advantage of not changing colour; but these are better adapted for entire sets than for separate teeth. Great improvements have been made in this art.

During these pioneer days, land settlement of immigrants was still the main occupation of the colony, money was scarce, and the few practitioners of health services found difficulty in making a living. William Dunlop, a British surgeon who first came to Canada with the army during the War of 1812, wrote at that time, 'Taller than most European women, slight and sallow, the women of the frontier weathered quickly. Hardly a woman of twenty could be found, who had not already lost half her teeth ...'[6] Dentists were very few, though occasionally one advertised in the press of towns like Kingston and Cobourg and at times travelled to lesser settlements for a day or two. Filling of teeth and provision of plates were not for the poor however; reference is made to a set of artificial teeth priced at £30, the equivalent in modern purchasing power of well over $1,000.[7] 'Pliers or tooth drawers' were used to pull teeth when the occasion demanded, and dentists and doctors were not alone in extracting them. Many a farmer built up a local reputation as a tooth puller.[8]

The distressing reality of toothache was the chief fact of dentistry as far as the pioneers were concerned. Complaints recur in the sparse literature of the times. In retrospect, the early availability and use of cloves seems rather surprising. Spice was one of the earliest commodities of international trade, and spices were being brought to the settlers on the New England coast at an early date; yet with the difficulties of transportation, one might not have expected to find evidence of their use by the early settlers in Canada. The first call for spices was to relieve the monotony of a limited, bland diet, but in time it was found that a piece of clove, shaped and fitted in the cavity of an aching tooth, would ease pain. Later, the oil pressed from cloves was used on a small fragment of absorbent material. For abscessed teeth, the pioneers also used sliced hot onions, placed in a sack and held against the cheek. An early Canadian recipe for cleaning teeth consisted of equal parts of orris root, charcoal, and whiting, pulverized together and applied by finger or brush. White of egg was recommended for canker sores.

Gunsmiths were recognized as expert, and very necessary, craftsmen in the early days, and many of them engaged in dentistry as a sideline. Percy Ghent of Toronto, a modern writer with the happy faculty of making history live with accuracy, recognized this dual facility in an article entitled 'A Christmas Eve Sleigh Ride (1833)':[9]

Have we heard about the Christmas present old Jock Stocking, the hatter, has bought for himself? No, well, for years, until yesterday, Jock hadn't a tooth in his head. But a month or so ago, he went to see the Frenchman, Isaac Columbus, the gunsmith of Caroline Street, to have a gun fixed. 'How are you going to eat the venison when you get it, with never a tooth to bite with?' says Isaac. 'You had better make me a set,' answered Jock, in a joking way. And Isaac did. They're as natural as life, and they work. Isaac can make anything.

In several instances, the records show that gunsmiths eventually became dentists. One of the most notable examples was the Martin family of Ottawa.

3
Late colonial period
1840-1859

Aldis Bernard crossed the border at the Niagara frontier in 1840. He was born on the shore of Lake Memphremagog, Quebec, in 1810 but at an early age was taken by his family to the southern United States. Evidently he served an apprenticeship with an American dentist and started practising about 1834. On his return to Canada, he spent a year trying to find a suitable place to establish a practice in the Niagara peninsula without success. Toronto, with a population of 12,000, was considered well supplied by two resident dentists. He continued his search to Montreal, where he practised until 1876, being one of the founders of the profession in the province of Quebec. At the time of his arrival in Montreal, which then had 40,000 inhabitants, there were three other dentists established in practice, namely Logan, Scripture, and John R. Spooner. Bernard was very active in municipal affairs, becoming mayor of Montreal in 1873.

One of the early dentists to establish practice, other than in the larger centres was G.V.N. Relyea. He was born in Albany, NY, and took lectures at the Albany Medical College in his spare time, while employed as a clerk. Later, he studied dentistry for a year with a practising dentist, and then practised on his own at several locations in New York State for a short time. After surveying the larger towns of Upper Canada, he settled in 1843 in Belleville (population then 2,500), where he practised until 1874. By his own statement, he had command of dental practice between Cobourg and Kingston. He spent two days every other week at centres other than Belleville. At these towns he had assistants (qualifications unknown) who extracted teeth, and he made the plates. Relyea was an astute businessman. In the fifties he learned about the invention of

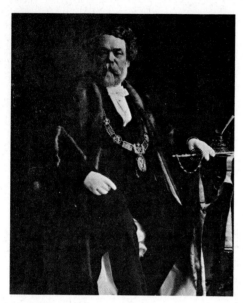

Aldis Bernard, Mayor of Montreal, 1873

vulcanizers, journeyed to New York, obtained the agency, and sold vulcanizers to dentists in Canada for a number of years. Later, he was active
in founding the profession formally in Ontario.

Until 1840, there is little evidence that Canadian youth exhibited
interest in learning to become dentists. Soon after that, however, the
number of dentists began to increase through apprenticeship training. For
the most part, the education was brief and rudimentary, and men started
out on their own with little knowledge or skill. Some settled down and,
gradually, towns of any size gained a resident dentist. Picton, Ontario,
seems to have been one of the earliest of the smaller towns to gain resident
dentists, as indicated in the 1860 advertisements placed in the Picton
Gazette by 'Dr' Fanning and Henry T. Wood. The latter was a self-trained
dentist who became one of the founders of the profession. Many of the
newly-trained men instead became itinerants throughout the country and
smaller municipalities. Often they travelled on foot with a back pack
containing the tools of their trade. Vulcanite came into general use as a
denture base during the late 1850s, one result being a rapid increase in
the number of travelling dentists who extracted teeth and made dentures
only. Perhaps an accurate case from the late 1860s will illustrate.

1868.   1868.

RELYEA,

DENTIST.

MR. RELYEA at the close of 1867, desirous to express his thanks to all who have employed him for the last twenty years. Gratified for the confidence placed in his professional ability for so long a period, it is his intention to avail himself of every modern improvement to please and benefit his patrons.

Owing to the gradual increase in business, and the demand on his constant personal services at the operating chair, he has found it necessary to engage a thoroughly competent mechanical dentist, who will now have the exclusive charge of that department.

A great deduction in the price of artificial teeth has taken place in consequence of the introduction of the rubber base, and thus the means of obtaining this very necessary addition to a pleasing personal appearance has come within the means af all.

Mr. Relyea takes pleasure in assuring those who, through fear of pain, have been deterred; that by means of the Nitrous Oxide Gas, he is daily extracting without pain; and if desirable, inserting new teeth the same day.

Testimonials to the safety, as well as the pleasing effects of this gas, are given below from the leading medical gentlemen of the Town.

TESTIMONIALS.

We the undersigned medical practitioners of this Town, from our knowledge of the chemical properties of the Nitrous Oxide Gas, give it as our opinion that it is a perfectly safe Anæsthetic, and do not hesitate to recommend our patients to avail themselves of its benefits in the extracting of teeth:

Robt. Stewart, M. D.   Rufus Holden, M.D.
D. E. Burdett, M. D.   Wm. Canniff, M.D.
Jas. Lister, M. D.   Wm. Hope, M. D.

For the further convenience of his patients' he has now for sale the safest, best, and most agreeable tooth powder, (in fact, as the ladies say, the use of it is a perfect luxury,) that can be made.

He has also a lotion for strengthening the gums and purifying the breath, and a cure for ague in the face, and toothache caused by cold.

An assortment of excellent tooth brushes, &c.,—indeed, every article required in the profession.

Belleville, Dec. 30, 1867.   22

Dental advertisement in the Belleville (Ontario) *Intelligencer*, 1868

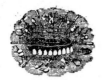

DR. G. W. FANNING,
Surgical & Mechanical Dentist,

WOULD respectfully announce to the Inhabitants of Picton, and surrounding
country, that he has opened an office on Main
Street, in the same building formerly occupied
by Dr, Relyea, where he may be consulted in
all cases relative to his profession.

ARTIFICIAL TEETH INSERTED ON
VULCANIZED RUBBER, &c.

☞ This material is considered one of the
greatest discoveries ever made in Mechanical
Dentistry. It is perfectly tasteless, and as
durable as gold. Cavities of the teeth will be
so filled as to prevent further decay and pain
for life.

ALL OPERATIONS WARRANTED.

DR. FANNING will insert teeth over roots,
if requested, so that patients will not require
to have the roots extracted.
                    G. W. FANNING.
Picton, 22nd Nov, 1860.   642

HENRY T. WOOD,
DENTIST,

BEGS leave to announce that he has
located in Picton, where he is
prepared to execute all work entrusted to him.
Teeth inserted on Vulcanise Base.
OFFICE: Next door to A. Bristol's store.
☞ **All work warranted.** ☜
Picton, June 21, 1860.   v12-6m-n48

From the Picton (Ontario) *Gazette*, 1860

Cicem Dorland was plodding along a back concession road northeast of Belleville on a cold winter day calling from farmhouse to farmhouse. He had a pack on his back which must have been heavy, for it contained a vulcanizer, forceps, a few instruments, and other materials for the making of dentures At one farmhouse he found a girl of fifteen years, who had been staying inside for several days. She had cavities between her two front teeth which ached when she went out of doors. By Dorland's own admission, her other teeth were good but his diagnosis was quick. He was invited to stay overnight and the following morning he extracted her upper teeth, without anaesthetic of any kind, took an impression in bees-wax, poured a model in plaster of paris, and produced a continuous gum denture with which the patient ate her supper. The vulcanizing was done on the kitchen stove. To the dentist of our time this whole procedure was about the worst service dentistry could offer, but in fairness to Dorland, it must be said that the patient was wearing this same denture in pristine condition on her seventy-fifth birthday. The patient was my mother.

By the 1850s, dentistry was being practised by four types of individuals.

1   Medical practitioners performed emergency services. Of necessity practically all physicians possessed a few pairs of forceps for extractions and by various means attempted to relieve pain for patients.

2   A few graduates of medical schools took some apprenticeship training and confined themselves to the practice of dentistry.

3   The flamboyant type of dental practitioner arrived in urban centres, preceded by extravagantly advertised claims. These men made generous use of handbills, testimonials and newspaper advertisements, claiming a perfection which today's dentist would find not only abhorrent but impossible.

4   An increasing number of men had served an apprenticeship of varying length with a dentist. At first, the indentureship was a loose arrangement, but gradually it became a rather severe legal contract between preceptor and apprentice. W. George Beers was to become the most outstanding Canadian dentist for a number of years. His indentureship, drawn up legally in 1856, reads as follows:[1]

On this day the ninth of December in the year of our Lord one thousand eight hundred and fifty six. Before us the undersigned Notaries Public duly commissioned and sworn in and for that part of the Province of Canada heretofore constituting the Province of Lower Canada residing in the City of Montreal in the said Province.

Personally came and appeared Mr. James C. Beers of the said City of Montreal Gentleman who for the good and advantage of his minor son William George Beers aged fifteen years on the fifteenth day of May last past declared to have bound and engaged and by these presents he doth bind and engage his said son now present and consenting as testified by his becoming a party to and signing these presents, to and with Charles M. Dickinson of the said city of Montreal, Esquire Surgeon Dentist party hereto and accepting of the said William George Beers as his covenant student and apprentice to the study and profession of Dentist for and during the term of four years, to be computed and reckoned from the twenty-second day of the month of November last past 1856 during all of which time the said William George Beers shall and will willingly serve the said Charles M. Dickinson obey his lawful commands do no hurt and damage to him in any manner howsoever neither see or suffer it to be done by others without giving instant information thereof to the said Charles M. Dickinson; shall follow his directions, attend regularly every day during the said period of said apprenticeship the surgery of the said Charles M. Dickinson and all and every the particular and general duties which may from time to time be assigned to him by the said Charles M. Dickinson; and finally shall demean himself towards the said Charles M. Dickinson as a good attentive and faithful student ought and is bound to do.

And the said Charles M. Dickinson for divers good and lawful considerations him thereunto moving and for and in consideration of the services so to be rendered by the said William George Beers doth hereby promise, bind and oblige himself to teach and instruct or cause or procure to be well and sufficiently taught and instructed the said William George Beers in and about all and every matter and branches connected with and touching and concerning the profession of a Dentist in so far as the said William George Beers has the capacity to take up and learn the same; and further should the said William George Beers conduct himself during the term of his present engagement to the entire satisfaction of the said Charles M. Dickinson he the said Charles M. Dickinson will allow him a sum of twelve pounds and ten shillings for each and every year of the said apprenticeship which said sum it is perfectly understood shall not be considered as a salary, but merely as an incentive to good behaviour on the part of the said William George Beers which can either be paid or retained by the said Charles M. Dickinson as he may think the said William George Beers deserving or not thereof; and in the event of continued misbehaviour or insubordination on his part it shall be optional with the said Charles M. Dickinson immediately to discharge the said William George Beers and cancel the present indenture without any notice whatever.

And it is hereby further agreed and understood by and between the said parties hereto that should the said Charles M. Dickinson give up the practice of his said profession either from ill health or otherwise at any time prior to the expiry of the term of the present engagement, he then shall have the privilege of either cancelling the present Indenture or of transfering them for the unexpired period through to his successor in which case all the Covenants and engagements herein entered into will be as binding and obligatory as if no such change or transfer had taken place. [An initialled marginal note to this paragraph reads 'With the consent of the said James C. Beers being first asked and obtained.']

And for the Execution of these presents the said parties hereto have respectively elected domiciles at their ordinary places of abode above mentioned.

Done and Passed at the said City of Montreal in the office of James S. Hunter one of said Notaries on the day, month and year first hereintofore written under the number one thousand nine hundred and twenty two and signed by the said parties hereto with and in the presence of us said Notaries these presents having been first read to said parties.

James C. Beers

William G. Beers

C. M. Dickinson

On a wall of the Faculty of Dentistry, Dalhousie University, Halifax, hangs a portrait of Dr Lawrence E. Van Buskirk, who is identified on a plaque beneath the painting as, 'The first man to administer an anaesthetic for a surgical operation in Canada.' Van Buskirk graduated in medicine from Columbia University in 1828. He practised medicine at Woodstock, NB, for five years and then after some study confined his practice to dentistry at Halifax, becoming the first permanent dental practitioner of repute in Nova Scotia. Hearing of the discovery of general anaesthesia by W.T.G. Morton, he went to Boston, learned the technique, returned to Halifax, and began extracting teeth with the use of ether. These facts are verified, particularly by D.M. Parker, a physician who, hearing of Van Buskirk's success in administering anaesthesia for extractions, requested his assistance. Parker wrote:[2]

Lawrence VanBuskirk, a dentist practising in Halifax, learned that ether was being used by inhalation in practical dentistry, visited Boston and familiarized himself with its use. On his return, having a case that required amputation of a femur, went to VanBuskirk's office and asked him to administer ether to him, as he personally would have some knowledge of its action. The next day, VanBuskirk administered ether, the limb was amputated.

It is to this operation that the plaque below Van Buskirk's portrait refers. The *Royal Gazette* for 16 February 1848 moreover contains the following statement: 'Dr L.E. Van Buskirk had made an inhaler and for the last year has used ether for over 100 extractions. Now that Chloroform has been used by doctors in Halifax, Dr Van Buskirk is using chloroform.'

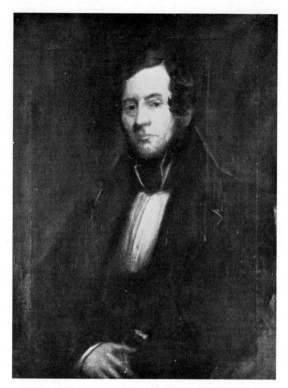

Lawrence E. Van Buskirk, first man to administer an
anaesthetic for a surgical operation in Canada

This latter statement places the advent of general anaesthesia by ether
in Canada to be early in 1847. Since Morton made his demonstration in
Boston only in October 1846, Van Buskirk must very quickly have
realized the great importance of the discovery. One or two other dentists
have claimed by inference to be the first to use general anaesthesia in
Canada. Of these J.H. Webster of Montreal has made the strongest
claims in the literature. However, at no place are dates stated, and for
the most part the claims consist of reminiscences by elderly men with
considerable confusion respecting dates. The fact that dentists were the
first to administer general anaesthetics in Canada is not disputed.

The Van Buskirk family were Knickerbocker Dutch, who came with
the Loyalists from New Jersey to New Brunswick. For a time during the

thirties, Lawrence and his brother George practised dentistry together at Saint John, and even after Lawrence went to Halifax he returned intermittently to practise with his brother. In a short history of early dentistry in New Brunswick, A.J. McAvenney vividly describes the administration of a general anaesthetic (presumably nitrous oxide) to a young lady, 'shortly after Dr Horace Wells, the American dentist, discovered surgical anaesthesia.'[3] This event places the administration of the first general anaesthesia for a surgical operation in Canada early in 1845, two years before the more sensational amputation. It is recorded that Lawrence Van Buskirk also was the first Canadian dentist to subscribe to a dental publication, the *American Journal of Dental Science*, in 1839.

Search of the literature indicates that W.H. Elliott of Montreal was the first dentist practising in Canada to make a contribution to dental journalism. In all, Elliott published 18 papers between 1842 and 1851. Originally he was an American dentist and is known to have practised in Plattsburg, NY, during 1845; afterwards he came to Montreal, probably in 1846–7, where he carried on a most successful practice until 1856, when George Van Buskirk of Saint John took it over. Before leaving the United States Elliott had published a number of papers, and it appears that his first contribution from Montreal occurred during 1847. An article by him and certainly from Montreal appeared in the January 1849 issue of the *New York Dental Recorder*. This article is of interest because it concerns his invention of an improved 'file carrier,' an instrument for operative dentistry, long since discarded but evidently in general use for many years. From the illustrations in the article, it appears to be a small edition of the fret-saw used by cabinet makers. It was used chiefly in separating teeth. Between 1849 and the early 1860s, articles appeared in American journals by such Canadian dentists as C. Brewster and George Beers of Montreal and G.L. Elliott of Toronto.

Some description of the practice of dentistry during the 1850s will indicate the stage of development. All operations were performed with hand instruments: another two decades would pass before the foot engine came into general use.[4] The greatest advance at this time was in the manufacture of artificial teeth. James A. Bazin of Montreal recalled that, 'Previous to this period most dentists had their own furnace for making "incorruptible" teeth, which resembled a split bean more than anything else.'[5] Manufactured artificial teeth now became available to dentists in continuous-gum and single-tooth forms.

The introduction of vulcanite in the late fifties re-oriented the whole practice of dentistry. Up to this time dentures had been built on metal base plates which were prohibitively expensive. Vulcanite made dentures available to most people. In the years to come a great number of other materials were introduced for use as base plates of dentures, the trade names of which are long since forgotten, but vulcanite held sway for nearly a century, until replaced by the acrylics.

Gold foil in many forms was the supreme filling, inserted in the prepared cavity with hand instruments. Cases are on record where the root canal was filled with gold as well as the cavity in the tooth. The beginnings of the use of leaf gold for filling teeth are unknown. Some historians date the use to the eighth century in Baghdad, but the supporting evidence appears inconclusive. Gold leaf in various forms was at any rate used by dentists in Europe during the eighteenth century. By 1812 one manufacturer in the United States specialized in beaten gold leaf for dental purposes. Definite evidence exists that Levi Spear Parmly used gold leaf in his practice at Quebec about 1815, and he was probably the first dentist in Canada to do so. Amalgam was known and used, but it was poor in quality and there was some fear of inserting mercury in the mouth. Dentists of repute seldom employed amalgam before the late 1850s, but the so-called quacks used it freely and often abused it – for example, by filling cavities in adjoining teeth without separation.

For extractions, the forceps were gradually replacing the key. The latter was a formidable instrument. There were many variations in design, but the one illustrated is typical in general. A mechanism somewhat similar to a miniature canthook grasped the tooth; the metal shaft and wooden handle gave the dentist sufficient leverage to wrest the tooth out of its socket. In Europe, the instrument was usually referred to as a 'key,' and there was a similar instrument known as the 'pelican.' In North America it was usually called a 'turnkey.' Forceps had been used to some extent before this period, but keys of various types had been preferred. Now they were being replaced by improved forceps that fitted the necks of teeth, although the key remained in use in outlying districts for many more years.[6]

Considerable variation existed in the kinds of instruments in the dental armamentarium. Each dentist designed and made his own instruments or had them made to his specifications. He may have copied an instrument used by another dentist or invented a new one. Instruments came to have the name of the inventor attached to them. Two innovations

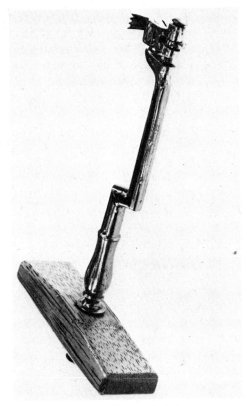

A turnkey – once a common dental
instrument, now a museum piece

in operative dentistry that appeared during the 1850s were spoon excavators for removing decay and Jack's chisels for cutting away enamel.

The manufacture of supplies to meet the need of dentists was still in
its infancy. In the United States, Samuel S. White began to practise dentistry in 1843 but retired in 1846 to devote his whole time to manufacturing, beginning with the production of artificial teeth and gradually
extending to other required dental supplies. In this period also the first
Canadian dental supply depot was established. Up to this time, and
probably for some time after, Canadian dentists were in the habit of
making trips at intervals to New York, Boston and Philadelphia to seek

new techniques and instruments. One such traveller was S.B. Chandler, who was born at Richville, NY, apprenticed at Ogdensburg, established practice at Port Hope, UC, in 1848, and later moved to Newcastle. He frequently made such trips and other dentists asked him to make purchases for them as well. As a result of this experience, he established the first dental supply house in this country, the Canadian Dental Depot, at Newcastle in the late 1850s. In 1883 he decided to devote his whole time to the dental supply business and moved his depot to Toronto.

The second Canadian supply business, the Toronto Dental Depot, was established in 1860 by C.H. Hubbard, who was born in London, England and came to Toronto in 1856 via New York. His original business was the manufacture of gold leaf, which he continued until his death in 1900. Gradually, he branched out into other dental supplies. This was the beginning of an inventive age in dentistry, and the establishment of dental depots made new kinds of supplies readily and conveniently available.

A notable event was the formation of the Halifax Visiting Dispensary Society in 1855.[7] The dispensary was supported by philanthropic citizens who paid an annual membership fee of 20 shillings each, and by a grant from the provincial government. Services were rendered at specified hours each day by 14 physicians, one dentist, and one apothecary. Patients who could afford to pay were charged a small fee, but for the most part treatment was free. The institution continued for several decades. This dispensary is the earliest recorded example of free dental services for the underprivileged in Canada.

On the Pacific coast, the earliest practitioners of dentistry were ships' surgeons, some of whom stayed in Canada for varying lengths of time. Despite considerable research, it is difficult to establish the first man to confine his practice to dentistry, but it appears to have been Joseph B. Haggin, a medical graduate who is said to have specialized in dentistry and practised in Victoria in 1858.[8] In this same year the first gold rush occurred, and other dentists arrived among the hordes of men crowding into the colony, chiefly from California. The second resident dentist appears to have been H.D. Longlaker, 'Surgical and Mechanical Dentist' in 1859.[9] By 1863, the city of Victoria had three dentists – G.W. Cool, S.M. Harris, and Thomas Walker.[10]

Some idea of the number of dentists practising by the year 1858 may be gained from municipal directories, which were freely published during these years for the larger centres (populations given in brackets). For

Nova Scotia five dentists were listed, all in Halifax (25,126). In New Brunswick seven appeared, three of them in Saint John (27,300). Canada East had not more than ten, with three in Quebec (51,000) and five in Montreal (75,000). In Canada West thirty-one dentists were listed, five at Toronto (50,000), four at Hamilton (29,000), and three at London (19,000). But these directories listed only dentists established in fixed practice.[11] Itinerant dentists in considerable numbers were travelling from place to place, making short visits to municipalities large and small. Any attempt to estimate the total number of dentists at that time would be difficult but the number was certainly small.

One dentist, whose name appears in most historical records of Canada, was W.H. Bown, a native of Brantford, Ontario, who travelled through rugged territory to the Red River Settlement (later Manitoba), arriving in 1863. He was a son of J.Y. Bown, MP for Brant from 1861 to 1873, and an intense patriot. Bown is referred to as the shadow of J.C. Schultz, a medical practitioner, who was prominent in founding the medical profession in Manitoba and was also active politically, becoming Lieutenant-Governor of the province in 1888. The Red River Settlement was made up of people of several nationalities, European immigrants, British, French, and the Métis, all of whom were highly independent in nature. Like other early practitioners, Schultz and Bown engaged in activities beyond the provision of health services, including fur trading and gold mining. Considerable resentment existed among the settlers respecting the introduction of legal measures from outside the settlement – even though the territory was recognized as British, nominally ruled through a monopoly held by the Hudson's Bay Company. Louis Riel became leader of the opposition. The first newspaper in the area, *The Nor'wester*, which was initiated in 1859, was bought by Schultz, and later sold by him in 1868 to his friend Bown.[12] Both Schultz and Bown used the newspaper to advance British aims and objectives, and hence received considerable credit in retaining the troubled territory as Canadian. During the Red River Rebellion when Riel was at the head of his self-styled provisional government and Bown editor of *The Nor'wester*, Riel demanded that Bown cease publishing a British proclamation and print material submitted by him. This Bown refused to do. As a consequence he was thrown in jail by Riel, but released by the military forces on their arrival. He was the first dentist in the area, and the first between southern Ontario and the Rocky Mountains.

Pierre Baillargeon was the first Canadian dentist to achieve notable

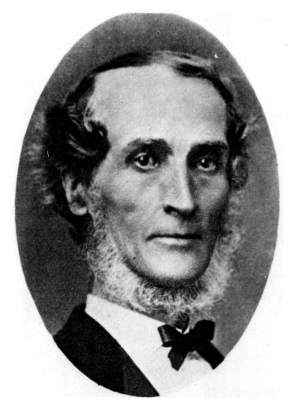

Senator Pierre Baillargeon

political recognition, being a member of the Senate from 1874 to 1891.[13] He was born at Crane Island, Quebec, graduated from Harvard University in medicine in 1840 and practised dentistry at Quebec City until his death in 1891. His name is the second on the Quebec Register of 1869, and he was an executive of the first Dental Association of the Province of Quebec. An interesting story is recorded respecting the Baillargeon family.[14] His mother had been left a widow with four small boys, and grew discouraged trying to bring them up. Then she had a dream that one would become an archbishop, two priests, and one a senator. All of it came true.

Changes in the colonies had their effect on the development of the profession. Perhaps the greatest change was in the numbers of people to be served. By 1852 the rapidly growing population of Canada West (952,004) had become greater than that of Canada East (890,261). The Act of Union of 1840, which had united Lower and Upper Canada as the provinces of Canada East and Canada West, had specified duties for the separate provincial administrations, and this led in time to confusion in seeking legislation for the profession. Until Bytown, re-named Ottawa, was selected as the capital of Canada by Queen Victoria in 1857, Parliament had roamed, meeting first at Kingston, then at Montreal, and then alternately at Toronto and Quebec City. Postage stamps were introduced in 1851 but until the railway came into being it still took five and a half days for a letter mailed in Montreal to be delivered in Toronto. Decimal currency was adopted in 1858. Until then the official currency was in pounds, shillings, and pence; but in fact many kinds of money were in circulation, varying in value from place to place. Dentists' fees were quoted generally in dollars, but often in sterling. The unsettled conditions contributed to the slow development of the dental profession.

Aldis Bernard of Montreal made what proved to be a premature attempt to obtain dental legislation during the 1840s. A bill for the incorporation of the College of Physicians and Surgeons of Lower Canada had been introduced in the legislature and Bernard, a man of influence, attempted to have additional clauses inserted for the regulation of dentistry. The bill became subject to acrimonious debate with accompanying delays, amidst which a ruinous fire occurred at the Court House. Papers, including the proposed clauses respecting dentistry, were destroyed. No further attempt was made to secure legislation for the control of dentistry for another twenty years.

Then, in 1860, Charles Brewster of Montreal sent a circular letter to all known dentists in Canada. His principal message was a protest against horrible dental exhibitions which were occurring at the time, but at the end he placed the following question: 'What is your opinion as to incorporating the dentists by Act of Parliament and obliging all those who in future may wish to practise in Canada, to pass a proper examination before a Board of Dentists?'[15] The replies to this question were unanimously favourable. Ways and means of carrying out the objective were investigated, until it was found that the Parliament of Canada would not consider the bill. Such legislation was under the jurisdiction of the provinces. As will be seen later, Brewster did not cease in his endeavour but for the while had to mark time.

The story of the Martin family illustrates remarkably well how some men became dentists during this period. Jean Paul Martin grew up on Ile Sainte-Hélène, the future location of Expo '67, where he became an expert mechanic and gunsmith. About 1840 he moved to Brockville, where the hunting was exceptionally good and his trade might be expected to prosper. His family consisted of four sons and four daughters. The sons – Alexandre (changed to Alexander), Olivier (changed to Oliver), Charles, and Joseph – all became dentists. In the early 1850s, when it appeared that Bytown was likely to be chosen as the capital, the family moved there, where the boys all engaged in their father's vocation. By 1860 Alexander and Oliver had turned to dentistry. For a time Charles worked in the railway shops at Belleville, Ontario, but returned and also took up dentistry in Ottawa. Joseph, the youngest, learned dentistry from his brothers and went to Hammond, Indiana, where he practised during his life. While the names of other dentists appear for brief periods, the three Martin brothers really established the profession in the Ottawa area. They were highly skilled craftsmen, and there is no indication that they served as apprentices in making the change to dentistry. Oliver in particular was a real student, as indicated by his well-used textbooks, which have survived. The brothers were highly independent by nature and, apart from collaborating for learning purposes, they conducted separate practices with very different characteristics. The oldest, Alexander, had as patients governors-general, prime ministers, including Sir John A. Macdonald, and other notables. Oliver was recognized as the leader in professional matters and had the largest practice, made up of the 'good' people of Ottawa. Charles's office at 24 Sussex Street was well-known by the local sporting fraternity. As a humorous after-dinner speaker, he was greatly in demand. According to the family he was much better as an entertainer than as a dentist; but he became an active leader as the number of dentists increased in the area, and as a consequence his name appears more often in dental literature than those of his brothers. For a long period, the three brothers were recognized as the foremost dentists of Ottawa. A son of Oliver, by the same Christian name, graduated from the Royal College of Dental Surgeons in 1890 and practised in Ottawa until his death in 1952. His son, Lawrence Melville, graduated from the same school in 1921 and also took up practice in Ottawa.

No account of this period would be complete without some description of the advertising by dentists. In comparison to the small size of the newspapers, many of the advertisements were large. Many portrayed a

194   ADVERTISEMENTS.

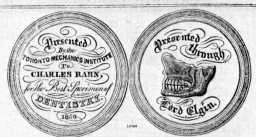

CHARLES RAHN,
DENTIST
TO HIS EXCELLENCY THE GOVERNOR-GENERAL.

RESPECTFULLY offers his services to the Ladies and Gentlemen of Toronto, who estimate the personal comforts of a Healthful Mouth, Sweet Breath, and Good Teeth.

The Professional experience of Mr. RAHN, acquired by many years constant practice in all branches of the Art, in addition to his intercourse with distinguished members of the Profession, warrants him in stating that his operations cannot be surpassed. He will PLUG THE TEETH to make them sound and stand the test of time ; INSERT TEETH not to be detected among the natural ones, and useful as beautiful; CLEANSE THE TEETH, RESTORE THE GUMS, AND IMPROVE THE MOUTH.

It is the intention of the Subscriber to execute his work in a manner so satisfactory to his patients as to render it unnecessary to the citizens of Toronto to resort for those professional services (which the health and happiness of every individual require) to those itinerating practitioners who are generally without responsibility, and who remain only for a few weeks in any one place; or to those inexperienced persons who congregate at the offices of migratory dentists, and commence practice after a few weeks' instruction.

Carious teeth will be stopped with GOLD or TIN-FOIL, without a resort to the destructive quackery of employing mercury in any of its amalgams.

REFERENCES:

Hon. Chief Justice Robinson,	Hon. Dr. Widmer,
Hon. Judge McLean,	Professor Gwynne,
Hon. L. H. LaFontaine,	" King,
Hon. R. Baldwin,	" Herrick,
Hon. H. J. Boulton,	" Nichol,
Rev. H. J. Grasett,	" O'Brien,
Rev. Dr. Lett,	" Richardson,
Rev. Dr. McCaul,	Dr. Hodder.
W. Proudfoot, Esq., Pres't. U.C. Bank,	Rev. Dr. Burns,
T. G. Ridout, Esq., Cashier U.C. Bank,	Dr. Rolph,
	Rev. Dr. Willis.

N.B.—Mr. R. begs to inform his friends who reside at a distance from Toronto, that he has never travelled the country, as they have been led to believe by some who assume his name, but may always be found at his Office,

CORNER OF BAY AND MELINDA STREETS, TORONTO.

An immodest advertisement in *Roswell's City of Toronto Directory*, 1850–1 set of artificial teeth, doubtless to attract attention. Particular ability was stated in superlative terms. Fees, sometimes with discounts, special techniques, and testimonials, were published. The advertisements of Charles Rahn of Toronto in 1850 seem today rather fantastic in the references offered: twenty-one names are given, including most of the notables of his time in the city. The inclusion of Baldwin and LaFontaine, government leaders of their day, seems incredible. Judgment must be related to the customs of the time and not to the ethical concepts of the present. Each age makes its own definition of customs, habits, and ethics.

Advancement of dentistry had been slow, at times distorted, and few indications existed of important changes which were about to take place. The number of dentists in the whole country was small, and among these only a comparatively few were able to make a full living from dentistry. Many had sideline occupations to supplement incomes, or practised dentistry as a sideline to more remunerative employment. Dentistry was expensive and only people of means could afford its services. Fortunately, among dentists there were a few, probably not more than half a dozen, who had foresight and vision which were to bear fruit in the near future. Important alterations were about to take place in the political sphere, and these men were ready to establish a place for dentistry within the concept of the new constitution.

4
Creation of a profession
1860-1869

The decade of the 1860s was one of great decisions in British North America. The colonies had till then been widely separated and sparsely settled, with little communication between them. By 1861, Canada had a population of 2,500,000. In Nova Scotia there were 325,000 people, New Brunswick had 250,000, Newfoundland 150,000, and Prince Edward Island some 80,000. With the increase in population the people became conscious of a new sense of maturity. After much hesitation, debate, and conferring among representatives of the colonies, the British North America Act was enacted in 1867 by the British Parliament and the Dominion of Canada was formed of Ontario, Quebec, New Brunswick, and Nova Scotia. At later dates, the other provinces joined in the confederation.

Circumadjacent to these political adjustments, social changes occurred. Reference in general literature to 'elegant Canadians' of the 1860s indicates that at least some of the people had attained success marked by a higher level in society. It would be a serious mistake, however, to interpret this advanced status as applying to more than a very few. Life for the vast majority of people was hard, organization scanty, money scarce, and the outlook precarious. Hardy pioneers were still clearing the bush in order to plant crops and establish frontier communities. It is a tribute to the faith and fortitude of our forebears that they tolerated the conditions which surrounded them. In their midst were high-minded men, albeit few, who endeavoured to bring about new order. With persistence, they worked through many discouragements to achieve improvements in the interests of future generations. Among them was Barnabus W. Day of

Kingston, who circulated a letter to known dentists in the province of Ontario in the fall of 1866, calling them to a meeting in Toronto early in January 1867.[1] Day was born on a farm near Kingston and is known to have been practising dentistry in Kingston during the late 1850s, having previously articled for six months with P.J. Sutton of Kingsbury, Quebec. While practising, he attended medical school at Queen's University, graduating in 1862 and afterwards continuing to practise dentistry.

Day did not claim originality for his idea. Charles Brewster of Montreal, to whom reference has been made in the previous chapter, had been in correspondence with him on the subject of incorporation. 'Dr Brewster realized that on account of the numerical strength of the profession in Upper Canada, the first steps should be taken there.'[2] The story circulated in following years was that Brewster's wife had relatives in Kingston and through this connection knew Day.

No one can be sure just how many dentists there were in Ontario at that time, for no professional regulation existed and many so-called dentists were scarcely entitled to the name. It is safe to assume, however, that the number was somewhat in excess of 100. The meeting was held at the Queen's Hotel, Toronto on 3 January 1867. Nine men were in attendance. As this was the first meeting called of Canadian dentists, it is appropriate to look briefly at these men.

Day has already been referred to. Curtis Strong Chittenden was born at Burlington, Vermont, obtained his training in New York State, and came to Hamilton in 1849, where he practised for forty years. During the 1850s he became a member of the Michigan State Dental Association and was elected its president in 1860; as a consequence, he was the only man of the group who knew something about professional organization.[3] Henry T. Wood came from New York State and practised in the town of Picton. He became known as a gentleman dentist who settled disputes. A more necessary type of man in the following years would be hard to imagine. Joseph Stuart Scott was a medical student at the time, who after graduation from Victoria Medical School later in the same year took up the practice of dentistry. F.G. Callender practised at Cobourg and while little is known about his origins, it is believed he came from New York State. John O'Donnell, who became the first secretary, practised at Peterborough. The others were A.D. LaLonde from Brockville, D.A. Bogart from Hamilton, and M.E. Snider from Toronto. Little is known respecting LaLonde and Bogart. It was said later that Snider was newly arrived in Toronto and attended the meeting out of curiosity. For some

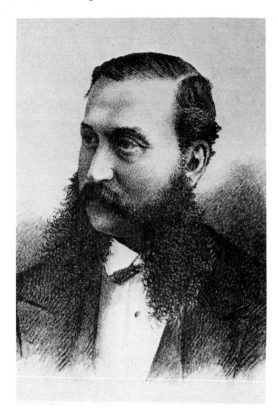

Barnabus W. Day, LDS, MD, father of dentistry in Ontario

unknown reason G.V.N. Relyea of Belleville, who was active in the cause, was not present at the meeting. Obviously the seven dentists practising in Toronto paid little, if any, attention to the letter sent out by a Kingston country dentist.

No minutes of the meeting have survived, but from published addresses, together with records following the event, a fairly clear picture of it is possible. Day was elected chairman, and stated that the purpose of the meeting was to find ways and means of securing legislation for dentistry. Probably through the influences of Chittenden, a decision was reached that it would be better first to organize the dentists and then to seek legislation. Four decisions were reached: first, that effort be made to secure legislation; second, that in order to attain this objective, it was first necessary to organize dentists; third, that a committee be appointed to draft a suitable constitution, and bylaws; fourth, that a meeting be called for the following July, at Cobourg to consider the report of the committee.

Some 31 dentists attended the Cobourg meeting, indicating an increased general interest. The main business was the adoption of the report on the constitution and bylaws, whereby the Ontario Dental Association came into being on 2 July 1867, the first organization of Canadian dentists.[4] The first decision reached by the newly created association was to seek legislation. A committee was appointed to seek advice and draft a bill for consideration at a meeting to be held the following January at Toronto.

The January meeting was held in St Lawrence Hall on King Street, the city's main place for important gatherings.[5] Confederation had become a reality and the first sesion of the Ontario Legislature was in progress at the Parliament Buildings on Front Street. It is evident that a great deal of work had been done in gaining support for legislation. A petition addressed to the Legislative Assembly had been circulated and signed by 68 dentists, 25 medical men, one judge, the mayor of Toronto, and a druggist.[6] The Medical Council had adopted a strong resolution in support. Two days were taken up with a discussion of the proposed bill. Some dentists opposed it on grounds that it was 'quixotic and immature' and, anyway, they did not want the government interfering with their private affairs. As a matter of fact, the opposition for the most part was made up of those who could not qualify under the bill's 'grandfather clause,' which granted recognition without examination only to those dentists who had been constantly engaged for a period of five years in established office practice. The insistence on 'established office practice' precluded, among others the 'tramp' dentists. Eventually the meeting adopted the proposed bill, and on the third day dentists and others of its supporters, numbering approximately 100, marched to the Parliament Buildings and the bill was introduced. Opposition by dentists continued during passage through the legislature, but with some minor amendments, the bill became law on 4 March 1868.[7]

During the six-month period between the Cobourg and Toronto meetings, the committee of the newly formed organization was very active. The securing of signatures on the petition required a great deal of time and effort. The drafting of an acceptable bill was a time-consuming matter for which advice was sought from every possible source. Probably through the influence of Relyea, the interest and co-operation of G.W. Boulter, MD, Member of the Legislature for Hastings County, was obtained. Boulter not only assisted in the drafting, but introduced the bill and persevered in piloting it through the legislature, finally succeeding on the last day of the session. No story of the legislation would be complete without due credit to Boulter.

This was the first Dental Act to be adopted anywhere in the world. The only legislation related to dentistry predating the Ontario Act occurred in the State of Alabama in 1841, when a section of three or four clauses was inserted in a medical bill. The Ontario Dental Act related to dentistry alone. In checking this point with the various state attorneys-general, it was found that the second such Act was adopted by the State of Ohio two months after Ontario's.[8]

The 1868 Act created the Royal College of Dental Surgeons of Ontario, with a Board of Directors elected by the members of the profession.[9] This body was granted full powers of licensing and regulating dentistry. The importance of the Act lay not only in that it gave the profession the right to govern itself, but in that it set a pattern for legislation in the other provinces. At various times there has been speculation as to how this type of dental legislation, which apparently does not exist in any other country, came into being. For dentistry, the reason appears clear. Legislation for medicine had already been enacted by the Parliament of Canada West in 1865, establishing the College of Physicians and Surgeons on a similar basis. This legislation was reaffirmed by the Ontario Legislature in 1868. In view of the fact that members of the medical profession assisted, probably with the same legal advice, in formulating the legislation for dentistry, it is reasonable to believe that the pattern already adopted for one profession was followed with minor variations. Indeed, a corporate body for the legal profession, the Law Society of Upper Canada, had been established as early as 1822, and has been continued by each successive Law Society Act to the present. The right of self-government by the professions has existed from the beginning in Canada and the principle has withstood the test of time. This freedom has, in a large manner, accounted for the rapid development not only of the dental profession but of all professions in Canada.

Dentists in the Province of Quebec quickly followed their Ontario colleagues. A meeting was held, with some 15 dentists present, on 2 September 1868 in Montreal, where the Ontario Act was reviewed clause by clause. The Dental Association of the Province of Quebec was initiated and a committee appointed to draft a constitution and bylaws. Aldis Bernard was elected president and W. George Beers secretary. A series of meetings of the association followed at which the main business was consideration of draft legislation for incorporation. It was thought expedient to follow the Ontario Act in so far as possible. An Act to incorporate the Dental Association of the Province of Quebec was enacted by the Quebec Legislature on 4 April 1869. There were several minor differences from the Ontario legislation; a notable one was that in Quebec the founding association was incorporated while in Ontario a new College was created, leaving the original association 'out in the cold.'

In the other two provinces, Nova Scotia and New Brunswick, efforts were made to secure legislation during 1869 without success. One phase of the difficulties faced was described by A.J. McAvenney of Saint John, NB, in an address several years later: 'In 1867 St John was honoured by having a dentist from Paris, Louis de Chiverie by name. Louis, for several years, hovered between St John and Halifax, taking in towns of New Brunswick and Nova Scotia. He was noted for his outdoor display ... He impressed himself so much on the members of the Nova Scotia Legislature that when Dr Allen Haley presented a bill to regulate dentistry in that province in 1869, it was rejected.'[10] As an editor, W. George Beers, never one to mince words, also referred to this event: '... But alas! what has poor Nova Scotia done that she should be afflicted with that little quintessence of quackery and rascality styled de Chevry, who it appears by the Acadian Recorder, recently appeared in Halifax in a sleigh drawn by four white horses, and so "lectured" a gaping crowd against the passage of a law in Nova Scotia incorporating the dental profession.'[11] The profession in these Atlantic provinces was to wait another twenty years for legislation.

The enactment of legislation in Ontario and Quebec constituted a great advancement, giving legal recognition to the dental profession. However, it was quickly discovered that existence of a law requiring practitioners to possess a licence and the implementation of that law were not one and the same thing. Custom and habit can create a law but they also can render a law ineffective. The Boards established under the Acts found themselves with the difficult task initially of separating those who qualified under the legislation from those who were not qualified, and then of controlling the activities of the unqualified as well as keeping the qualified in order. At times, the difficulties seemed almost insurmountable. Unfortunately, on many occasions an individual whom the Board refused to recognize was granted a licence by decree of the legislature. Such action ceased gradually, and terminated only over several decades.

Being a member of a Board proved to be an arduous task, demanding a great deal of time. Some of the cases received considerable newspaper publicity, which did not always aid the Boards' endeavours – although at other times it was helpful. In 1870, for example, an individual named C.H. Stewart hung out his shingle in Montreal and attracted considerable attention by his low prices and marvellous promises. Documents and a photograph produced at a meeting of the Quebec Board identified Mr Stewart as a dentist named C. Sill who had run away from Pittsburgh with a woman named Kate Fry, leaving a wife and several children in a state of destitution, and showed that Kate Fry was living with him as his wife. A Montreal newspaper got hold of the circumstances and made Stewart's name still more notorious by publishing the following 'free lance' poem.

Ah! Dr. Sill to run away,
  And leave your 'better fraction,'
And olive-branches, was, we think,
  A very *silly* action.

In fact, we are inclined to say,
  – Now, please don't shed our blood, Still –
That, in the language of the South,
  You are a precious 'Mud-*sill*!'

A dentist, too – well hold your jaw; –
  Canadian skies beneath,
By *gum*, there are some folks who dare
  To cast it in your teeth.

Kate Fry! – such an appropriate name,
  But surely meets our eye,
Were you sick of domestic broils
  That you preferred a *Fry*?

Consistent too, until the last,
  Your *nom-de-guerre* shows true art,
For you've converted Mrs Fry,
  Into a Mrs *Stew*-art.

Ah! Doctor Sill, ah! Doctor Sill,
  This is no theme for laughter,
Take care lest *Fry*-ing be your fate
  In this life *and hereafter*.

The poetry is bad but the result proved efficacious. After such publicity the Board rejected Stewart's application on the sole grounds of immoral character. So satisfied was Stewart of the position of the Board that he at once retired from practice.

From the present point of view the examiners appointed by the Board performed their work with competence. The task was a difficult one, in that just about the only available training was by apprenticeship. A number of graduates from medical schools were registered, but for the first two years after the Acts only one graduate from a recognizable dental school appears on the provincial registers – H.H. Nelles of London, Ontario, who graduated from the Baltimore College of Dental Surgery in 1860.[12] As time went on, the most frustrating part of the legislation was the provision that (in Ontario) persons 'who have been constantly engaged for five years and upwards in established office practice, next preceding the passage of the Act' were entitled to licence upon furnishing satisfactory proof, and without examination. In Quebec, the required time was two years. Rather elaborate affidavit forms were formulated, to be sworn by a minister, a medical practitioner, and a well-recognized citizen to the effect that the applicant was known by them to have fulfilled the stated condition. Initial decisions were easily reached, based on the affidavits and knowledge of the individuals, but as applicants continued to present themselves in possession of the required affidavits over the next twenty years, the process became rather ridiculous.

Beginning in the 1860s and until the end of the century, the name of W. George Beers of Montreal was a dominating one in the life of the profession. It is well to pause in order to summarize, for no history of Canadian dentistry during the following four decades could be compiled without repetitive reference to this man. At the time of his death, in 1900, a Montreal daily newspaper described him as 'a well-known dentist, a fearless patriot, a famous athlete, an efficient militia officer, and a much respected citizen.' Beers was born in Montreal in 1841, served his apprenticeship with a dentist named Dickinson, and practised in that city all his life. He was the first secretary of the Quebec Association, later becoming president. He served his profession in innumerable ways, as an editor, as dean of the first dental school in Quebec, and as a public adviser on all matters related to dentistry. His reputation as a public speaker was great, both within and without dentistry. As a sportsman he gained a tremendous reputation, particularly as an authority on lacrosse. He carefully watched the play of Indians, to whom the game originally belonged, and drafted the first set of rules. On two occasions he took lacrosse teams on

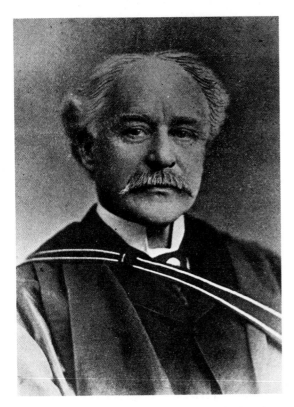

William George Beers, DDS, editor, dean, and a founder
of Canadian dentistry

his own to England, where a series of games were played, including one
before Royalty. His patriotism led him into the militia and he served
during the Fenian raids, retiring with the rank of captain. He wrote
widely, not only on dentistry but also on sports and patriotism, and was
published both in Canada and the United States. Beers was a great man
of his era. Perhaps an author's personal note will not be out of place. In
the periodicals and books coming into my home during the year 1967,
George Beers was the subject of six articles, two in Centennial books, two
in newspapers, and two in institutional publications. In any walk of life,
not many men will receive such tribute so long after death.

Here, our interest is in his establishment in 1868 of the *Canada Journal of Dental Science.* He started it with his own resources. Two short-
lived efforts in dental journalism preceded this event. In 1854, there had

been a few issues of a publication entitled *The Family Dentist*, edited by
S.S. Blodgett of Brockville, Ontario; and the *Journal of the Times* had
appeared irregularly at Halifax between 1858 and 1860, published by
Paine and Macallister.[13] In reality, Beers' was the first dental journal in
Canada. He was a splendid reporter, and it is from this source that most
of the historical information is to be obtained for the period. Potential
subscribers were few in number, however, and financial difficulties soon
arose. The *Journal* was first published in Montreal, beginning in June
1868, then in Hamilton where C.S. Chittenden acted as assistant editor
for a period, and finally moved back to Montreal. The *Journal* appeared
monthly until October 1871, but the last issue of Volume 3 did not appear
until May 1872. Only four issues of Volume 4 appeared and these were
widely separated, the last being in August 1879. But Beers was persistent.
He attempted to obtain financial support in all possible ways, including
assistance from the existing associations, with no success. Without question, he drained his personal finances in order to publish a journal in the
interests of the profession.

CANADA JOURNAL

OF

DENTAL SCIENCE,

Editors and Proprietors,

W. G. BEERS,
C. S. CHITTENDEN,
R. TROTTER,

—•◦•—

VOL. 1.

—•◦•—

HAMILTON,

1869·

Title page of Canada's first true dental journal

In Ontario, almost immediately after the legislation was enacted, pressure developed for the establishment of a dental school. The Board established a committee to investigate the feasibility of such action. In October 1868 the committee reported that 'we consider it impracticable and inexpedient therefore not judicious to start such an institution at the present time.' George L. Elliott, a member of the Board, was a member of the committee and signed the report, making it unanimous. Yet even then he must have had other negotiations under way, for almost immediately a rather elaborate announcement appeared of the establishment of the Canada College of Dentistry with Elliott as dean. The faculty was named and the course described; the first session was to run from 1 December 1868 to 1 March 1869, with a tuition fee of $50. Statements appear later that the Board of the College had approved the course and agreed to recognize the graduates, but no such agreement is to be found in the Board minutes. Nor is much else known today of the school. Seven students attended the first course, and at least one dentist claimed in newspaper advertisements to be a graduate of the Canada College of Dentistry. Dr. D.V. Peacock of Brockville also mentioned the college in a large street sign in front of his office. But no address in Toronto for the school was stated in the announcement, and it has not been possible to find its location. The minutes of the Board reveal very little detail about the school except that there was heated controversy over it. A year and a half after he signed the report recommending against a dental school, Elliott

ESTABLISHED
1867.

DENTISTRY.

ESTABLISHED
1867.

D. V. BEACOCK,

Licentiate of the Royal College of Dental Surgeons of
Ontario, and Graduate of "Canada College
of Dentistry."

TEETH EXTRACTED WITHOUT PAIN

By the use of Nitrous Oxide Gas. Over 10.000 persons
have taken it in my Rooms since 1867 without
a single accident.

Teeth filled with Gold, Silver, Felt Foil, and all the
more modern plastic fillings.

Full Sets of Teeth inserted from $10 upwards.

Try D. V. BEACOCK'S

Aromatic Enamelene for Cleansing the Teeth.   Over 1.000
Bottles sold during 1878.

A dental office sign from 1880. Beacock graduated from the first Canadian dental school, a short-lived private institution in Toronto published a rather elaborate and extended explanation, but undoubtedly presented only one side of the matter while little was recorded on the other. The school was not a financial success. Its importance lies in that it was the first effort in Canada to establish a dental school and the only effort ever made in the country to operate a private dental school for profit. While Elliott claimed in 1870 that the Canada College of Dentistry was still being sustained, little is heard of it thereafter.

In July 1869 the Ontario Board, reversing its previous decision, agreed to establish a dental school immediately. The action appears to have been a hasty one, probably influenced by the controversy with Elliott, who was a member of the Board until 1870, when he was not re-elected at the annual meeting of licentiates. The Board decided not to name a dean, but appointed F.G. Callender, a reputable practitioner at Cobourg, as professor of operative dentistry and J. O'Donnell of Peterborough as professor of mechanical dentistry, and arranged for the basic sciences to be taught by the medical schools. The course was six months in length beginning October 1; the fee was $100. The Board granted a sum not to exceed $300 to support the school.

Two students presented themselves and completed the six-month course – Benson Gilbert of Belleville and James Woods of Sarnia. At the close of the session, the Board was faced with a deficit of approximately $125, and in July 1870 a resolution was passed cancelling the arrangement. Today the amount appears small to prompt such decision, but money at that time was a scarce commodity of which the Board had little, the value of a dollar was much greater, and the future did not appear bright. The effort must have proved costly to Callender, who moved to Toronto from Cobourg to take his position, and for O'Donnell, who travelled back and forth from Peterborough to teach when travelling was a comparatively slow and uncomfortable process. After these rather disastrous attempts to establish a school, no further effort was made until 1875.

The difficulties of implementing the legislation and instituting formal education are difficult to comprehend for our present-day generation. There were in the seventies some first-class men who worked assiduously for advancement, but there also existed a class of men who attempted in every way to discredit altruistic efforts. Henry T. Wood described them in a later address, stating that his story was not coloured in any way.[14]

Men who went about the country ignorantly and presumptuously talking dentistry to the curious crowds which gathered to listen to them, and sometimes before the victim was aware of his intentions the dirty fingers of a dental vagabond would enter a rustic's mouth and many a good molar would be doomed. Then would come the professional advice. 'Several teeth must be pulled and others should be filled.'

As a rule, this would occur in the country and among the farmers who had large families, and the 'doctor' had a keen eye in business when he learned one of the sons of the house was suffering from toothache. 'Well,' said he, 'It is a lucky thing for you that I've come round here today. We'll soon pull out all the ache, and put the teeth of the whole family in good shape.'

'But,' the farmer would say, 'what about the cost? When there are so many teeth to be filled and extracted seems to me you ought to make some reduction in your prices. Do you?'

'Of course I do,' says the doctor; 'there will be no trouble on that point. My price is twenty-five cents for each silver filling, and ten cents for pulling a tooth. Why, if you went to town to have this job done it would cost you from fifty to seventy-five cents for silver fillings, and twenty-five cents for having a tooth pulled. Sometimes when I've a lot of work to do for one family I fill six or eight teeth for one dollar, and I don't suppose the whole job here will cost more than five or six dollars. So now, if you say the word, we will bring our tools in and begin right after dinner.

'Of course you'll feed the horse and give us our dinner in the bargain? Here is my assistant. I generally have some one to help me. You see I can take a smart young man and learn him the trade in six weeks. Now just look at this young man. This is his fourth week, and he can fill a tooth, just as well as I can, only not so quick. Say, farmer, you ought to have one of your boys learn the trade. It only takes about six weeks and the cost is only $100.00 and he will come out a first-class dentist.'

At the risk of some repetition, it is well to keep in mind the type of practice in the 1860s. As explained earlier, the introduction of vulcanite prompted a great increase in the practice of dentistry. Porcelain teeth were originally manufactured with long straight pins for soldering to the metal base plates. Dentists now bent these pins for retention in vulcanite; the 'footed pin,' while a small change, was considered a great advance at the time. Dental chairs were changing: the first ones were simply straight-backed kitchen chairs, to which a primitive head rest was added eventually. Later, a dentist would sketch out his needs and call on a cabinetmaker to build an upholstered chair specially for him. These chairs were comfortable for the patient, if not for the operator. The first iron chair, with movable back and seat, came into use during this period. Gold foil was the supreme filling. It was inserted by hand pressure until 1861, when the hand mallet was introduced. Five years later the automatic mallet was invented. Both were welcome aids. The control of saliva was one of the great problems: although napkins of various types, duct compressors, tongue holders, and other appliances had been introduced, they were found to be only partially successful. In 1864 C.S. Barnum, a dentist in New York, invented 'rubber dam' and presented it to the dental profession. The need was great and Barnum was showered with recognition in the form of gifts, money, and medals from dental societies and individuals.

Amalgam was used freely by the so-called 'tramp dentist' but up to this point had made slow progress among the reputable practitioners owing to its poor quality. During this decade, however, improved types became available and its value was recognized. A small-sized amalgam war broke out in the late sixties between H.M. Bowker, a Montreal dentist, and George Beers, which attracted considerable attention and continued into the early 1870s. Bowker published his articles in the *Canada Medical Journal*, wherein he resurrected arguments against the use of amalgam which were dusty with negated age.[15] Beers refuted the statements with adequate proof. The articles continued until the editor of the *Canada Medical Journal* refused to publish more, whereupon Beers had the last word in his own *Canada Journal of Dental Science*.[16] Many other minor improvements occurred, but the pain of toothache was often surpassed by the pain of extraction.

The beginning of organization by dentists had occurred. As already observed, the Ontario Dental Association and the Dental Association (Société Odontotechnique) of the Province of Quebec were organized before any dental legislation existed. The Ontario Dental Association achieved its prime objective in obtaining the legislation, and unfortunately for the association, the efforts of the initial professional leaders became almost wholly taken up with the new Royal College of Dental Surgeons of Ontario. Dissension arose within the ODA and under the leadership of A.C. Stone, of London, a second organization, the Ontario Society of Dentists, was formed in 1868. Through the tact and diplomacy of a few, however, the two societies united in the following year. At the union meeting, held in Belleville in July 1869, a definite decision was reached that only one provincial organization should exist, but that in such a large province local dental societies should be formed, and efforts were bent in that direction. According to a statement made at that meeting, dentists in the Bay of Quinte area had been holding meetings for some time. Since

Day, Relyea, Wood and Callender (all originators of the ODA) practised in this area, it appears reasonable that they were in fact meeting previous to the first gathering called by Day in January 1867. In any event, the Quinte Dental Society became the first local dental society to be organized formally, in August 1869. In November of the same year the Western Dental Society was organized at Chatham with A.C. Stone of London as the moving spirit, and during the same year the Hamilton District Dental Society was organized, C.S. Chittenden being the leader. At this point, the effort appeared to peter out. It had been anticipated that Toronto, having the largest concentration of dentists would give leadership and an effort was made in 1870, but without success. Toronto delayed another twenty years before organizing a local society. The Montreal Dental Society was organized in 1871, the first local dental society in Quebec.

Jacob Neelands of Lindsay, Ontario, became noted for his early use of nitrous oxide for general anaesthesia in extracting teeth. Neelands began practice at Lindsay in 1861, after serving an apprenticeship of a year with his brother, T. Neelands, at Port Hope, and was still practising in 1928 at the age of 90. For many years he was known as Ontario's Grand Old Man of Dentistry. During his time he had many indentured students, several of whom gained prominence in the profession later. All spoke in glowing terms of him as a dentist.

Reference is sometimes made to Neelands as being the first to use nitrous oxide as an anaesthetic in Canada and he probably was in his own area. The question of priority in its use is difficult to determine because any decision would be based on fragmentary evidence. Horace Wells of Connecticut had conceived the idea of using nitrous oxide for surgical anaesthesia in 1844. It appears that a rather long period would have elapsed between its use by Wells and the 1860s when Neelands is reputed to have begun using it. The earliest reference found to its apparent use in Canada is in fact, as noted in Chapter 3, by the Van Buskirk Brothers in the mid-forties. Some evidence exists that gas (N_2O) anaesthesia was used by Montreal dentists prior to the 1860s, but names of individual users and exact dates have not been established. More definite evidence exists that H.H. Nelles of London was using nitrous oxide at the same time or before Neelands, and others, including J.B. Meacham of Brantford, laid claims to early use.

Study of the situation reveals that there was considerable difficulty both in obtaining satisfactory gas and in devising a method of administration. Neelands manufactured his own gas and devised equipment for administration which overcame the difficulties. For this he received and deserved great credit. Furthermore, he made his methods known to other dentists at a time when secrecy of techniques played a real part in dental practice. Dentists, then as now, rapidly seized new improvements to practice, particularly those for the relief of pain.

On the west coast, meanwhile, gold was exercising its eternal attraction. Initial discoveries along the lower Fraser and Thompson rivers led prospectors further north into the Cariboo country, and with the finding of gold in quantity there in 1862, thousands of men flocked to the area from distant places. Among them were an undetermined number of dentists. They probably came more to gain riches than to engage in practice, but some of them did provide dental service. Of these the main individual was William Allen Jones, a black dentist, originally from England, who made his way via the West Indies and California to Barkerville, the central mining town. In the *British Columbia Directory* of 1877–89, Jones is listed as a miner, but in recognition of his professional skills he had the distinction of being the first person registered under the British Columbia Dental Act, enacted in 1886. During recent years, Barkerville has been restored as a tourist attraction. Mainly through the efforts of L. King Grady, a Vancouver dentist, on behalf of the British Columbia Dental Association, Jones's dental office has been refurbished with the dentist and his patient present in manikin.

The decade of the 1860s was a momentous one nationally: a federation consisting of four provinces was created. Dentistry also made substantial progress, being recognized by professional acts in two provinces. By the end of 1870, there were 163 qualified dentists registered in Ontario and 37 in Quebec. But the picture was not completely bright. The first census taken in 1871, reported a population of 1,620,851 for Ontario and 1,191,516 for Quebec. The ratio of dentists to population was by no means favourable. On the other hand, public appreciation of the services that dentists were prepared to render was low; in fact, many dentists had to engage in money-making sidelines in order to ensure a living. Glowing stories of the professional celebrations held at the time of the enactment of dental legislation were current for many years after the event. Dentists of that time thought their troubles solved by law. Soon, however, the leaders of the profession discovered that privileges granted brought increased responsibilities, and if advancement was to be attained dentists themselves would have to achieve it.

5
Formal education
1870-1879

By the 1870s the eastern half of what is now Canada was well beyond its pioneer days. The typical Canadian of the period was a countryman, living on a farm, in the bush, or in a fishing village along the coast. Some nine cities, with population over 10,000, had developed by the time of the 1871 census. The three largest were Montreal, with a population of 129,822, Quebec, with 59,699, and Toronto, with 59,000. Saint John was the fourth largest with 41,325; Halifax, Hamilton, and Ottawa were in the twenty thousands, while London and Kingston had 18,000 and 12,407 respectively. Winnipeg had 241 persons. Already, the strong trend towards urbanization had begun which has continued to the present. In 1871, 80 per cent of all Canadians were classified as rural; by 1881 this figure had declined to 74 per cent. The population of the whole country in 1871 was 3,687,257, which increased to 4,324,810 by 1881.

Brick houses were replacing frame ones and every city had its mansions elaborately furnished. All towns worthy of the name possessed gas lighting, but the streets were as muddy as ever. Inventive minds were at work producing many improvements in the style of Canadian life. One such innovator was Alexander Graham Bell who invented the world's first telephone of practical use at Brantford, Ontario, in 1874. Lumbering was an important economic industry; mining was developing rapidly, and manufacturing, particularly of farm machinery, was well established.

After considerable negotiation, the province of Manitoba joined the Canadian federation in 1870. On 20 July 1871, one year later to a day, British Columbia became Canada's sixth province, and in 1873 Prince Edward Island came into formal union, thus creating one country 'A Mari

Usque ad Mare.' Between the provinces of Manitoba and British Columbia lay a vast area referred to as the North-West Territories, recognized as a part of Canada.

    A few selected items from dental records for 1871 may give some idea of matters of concern at that time. The Quebec Dental Society passed a resolution stating that 'all dental advertisements were unprofessional which drew attention in any way to special methods or modes of practice.'[1] Later during the same year the Ontario Board, at the behest of the Ontario Dental Society, cancelled the licence of S.J. Sovereign of Hamilton, who had become a notorious advertiser; but upon legal advice it withdrew the action.[2] These are the first recorded actions against advertising, a matter of concern for the next half century. At the second meeting of the Montreal Dental Society, an endeavour was made to establish a measure of control over non-paying patients. Decision was made to open a 'Black Book' in which would be entered the name and address of each 'dead-head' patient, and each member of the Society was to have a copy.[3] How practical this action proved to be is not recorded, but in modern terms it appears like an early attempt at credit rating. Exemption from jury service for dentists was a subject of much discussion which continued for several years, until granted. Following some debate, Beers stated in an editorial that while it was premature to establish dental hospitals, it would be 'highly desirable to have a dental department in connection with all general hospitals.'[4] The most absorbing activity in time and effort was the search for means of dealing with men practising without a licence. Great effort had gone into the securing of legislation and a tendency existed, among the rank and file of dentists, to think that the answer to all problems lay in seeking legislative amendments granting more powers to the profession.

    Very early, however, the leaders in dentistry realized that an Act did not automatically make a profession – legislation was only an initial advance toward professional stature, and constructive progress depended upon the efforts of dentists themselves. This was an important step forward. The first effort that followed was an attempt to find a way of securing adequate recompense for the dentist so that he could render his patients a service of good quality. At a meeting of the Quebec Dental Society in 1870, George Beers stated the matter tersely: 'If we consider dentistry a mere trade, then let us agree to work for a little over cost as the shoemaker who makes our shoes; but if a profession, let us charge for our brains.'[5] The difficulties faced lay, in the main, in two existing conditions. First, a considerable number of competent men were in dentistry, but probably the majority of practitioners were what were known as 'cheap dentists.' The well-qualified dentist found it necessary to charge two dollars for a gold-foil filling of good quality, while the cheap dentist inserted a filling of little value for seventy-five cents. The public suffered, and dental practice was downgraded. Second, the public in general had very little appreciation of dental services. Both conditions, in various forms, will have a familiar ring to the ears of at least the older dentists of our own period. The point is that they were realized early in the life of the profession.

Another factor which inhibited the development of dentistry for several decades was professional narrow-mindedness. Dentists vigorously protected the 'secrets' of their practice. Pupils were indentured with solemn formality, whereby the innocent student was legally bound not to open an office within one hundred miles of his preceptor, nor to reveal to rival dentists the 'secrets' he might learn in his preceptor's office or laboratory. Techniques were more important and personal than bank accounts. As a result of this attitude, any proposals for co-operation, association, or reform were met with repulsion. This attitude improved somewhat with the adoption of legislation, but its eventual disappearance was discouragingly slow. Meanwhile the development of true scientific organizations was deterred. As mentioned previously, a few dental societies were formed on other than the provincial level, but it was much later before society programs revealed 'secrets' or freely offered presentations of a true scientific nature.

Indentureship training was subject to many abuses and served to multiply the existing problems in many respects. The better practitioners took great care both in selecting a student and in training him, but other dentists, greater in number, simply used indentured students to their own advantage. Pressure developed again in Ontario for the establishment of a school. The Ontario Board was hesitant after the failure of two schools in Toronto, but the subject came under discussion at each meeting. Amendment to the Dental Act was secured to strengthen the hands of the Board in respect to education. At the same time, an amendment was sought to permit the granting of doctorates by the Royal College of Dental Surgeons of Ontario. This request was refused by the Legislature on the grounds that only a university could confer degrees.

Then the Board endeavoured to obtain some form of affiliation with a university and requested the Senate of the University of Toronto to establish a curriculum and examination in dental science, pointing out that

Harvard University had organized a dental department in 1867, leading to the degree of Doctor of Dental Medicine, and that the California State University had taken similar action, and was conferring degrees of Doctor of Dental Surgery. (The first dental school in the world, the Baltimore College of Dental Surgery, had been established in 1840. By the 1870s, other schools had been organized in the United States, but Harvard was the first to be under university jurisdiction.) The University of Toronto refused. It appears that lengthy discussions then took place with Queen's University, Kingston, but again with no favourable end result.

The matter of affiliation with a university was not wholly a question of whether or not dentistry should be recognized as a university discipline. A strong public argument that prevailed for many years against subsidization of the education of doctors and lawyers at a provincially-supported institution was that, once the students had qualified with public aid as members of lucrative professions, the public would have to pay over again for their services. At the same time, many dentists were anxious to secure the prestige of the title, 'Doctor,' and irritated that there was no way to obtain it legally in Ontario. Under the Act, the Board had power to grant no more than a Licentiate of Dental Surgery (LDS), sometimes mistakenly referred to as a degree. A few medical graduates who practised dentistry used the doctoral degree, and so did some Canadians who had graduated in the United States, for a number of independent dental schools there conferred doctorates without any university affiliation. But in Canada, only universities could grant degrees. From the beginning, many dentists freely used the doctoral degree to which they had no inherent right. This situation continued until 1889, after the Toronto school to be described next was affiliated with the University of Toronto.

In July 1875, the Ontario Dental Society, meeting in Hamilton, adopted a strong resolution requesting the Ontario Board to establish a school of dentistry in Toronto and 'to aid it by such appropriation of funds as in their judgement may be expedient.'[6] The quoted part of this resolution was all-important, because the main difficulty was financial. During the same month the Board took action. Two teachers were considered sufficient and the Board appointed J.B. Willmott and Luke Teskey. In view of the financial experience in operating the previous school, a carefully worded document was drafted, setting forth the conditions under which the school was to operate.[7] To summarize it, the first course of four months was to begin 3 November 1875; the two lecturers were to divide stated subjects between them; an infirmary was to be

First· Annual Announcement

OF

𝕿𝖍𝖊 𝕾𝖈𝖍𝖔𝖔𝖑 𝖔𝖋 𝕯𝖊𝖓𝖙𝖎𝖘𝖙𝖗𝖞

TORONTO.

Established under Authority of the Statutes of Ontario 35 vic. cap 34
by the

ROYAL COLLEGE OF DENTAL SURGEONS OF ONTARIO

SESSION OF 1875-6.

BOARD OF DIRECTORS AND EXAMINERS.

C. S. CHITTENDEN, L.D.S., President.
HENRY T. WOOD, L.D.S., Treasurer.
J. B. WILLMOTT, D.D.S., M.D.S., L.D.S., Secretary.
F. G. CALLENDAR, L.D.S., Registar.

L. CLEMENTS, L.D.S.   S. ZIMMERMAN, D.D.S., L.D.S.
C. P. LENNOX, L.D.S.

FACULTY OF INSTRUCTION.

J. B. WILLMOTT, D.D.S., M.D.S., L.D.S., Lecturer on Operative
and Mechanical Dentistry, Dental Pathology, Chemistry and
Materia Medica.

L. TESKEY, L.D.S., Lecturer on Anatomy, Physiology, Dental
Histology and Dental Surgery.

CLINICAL INSTRUCTORS AND DEMONSTRATORS.

F. G. CALLENDAR, L.D.S.   R. G. TROTTER, L.D.S.
M. E. SNIDER, L.D.S.   L. TESKEY, L.D.S.
S. ZIMMERMAN, D.D.S., L.D.S.   H. HIPKINS, L.D.S.

LECTURE ROOM AND INFIRMARY: 46 CHURCH STREET, TORONTO.

First announcement of the School of Dentistry, Toronto – eventually the University
of Toronto Faculty of Dentistry

opened for the gratuitous treatment of diseases of the teeth, with one of seven stated dentists to be present each morning; budgets of $150 for rent and $250 for furnishings were voted; the student fee was to be $100, which was to be used by Willmott and Teskey in operating the school; and there were to be eight applicants for the course before the school was started. In reality, Willmott and Teskey were granted $400 by the Board and asked to operate a school. The Board exercised considerable care to avoid responsibility for any deficits which might occur. These terms became subject to serious controversy within the profession at a later date. Money values of the time are not to be judged in modern terms: Timothy Eaton was offering bargains of a spool of thread for one cent and men's neckties at five cents each. The sums involved were in fact substantial.

The establishment of the school at Toronto was the most important event to take place in Canadian dentistry during the period from 1870 to 1890. The school became known as the Royal College of Dental Surgeons, ever to be confused with its creator, the Royal College of Dental Surgeons of Ontario.[8] The Board was very careful to make the money granted the final amount and to place the responsibility for financial success on the shoulders of Willmott and Teskey. The two men succeeded, academically as well as administratively. It is well to briefly observe them.

James Branston Willmott was born in June 1837 in Halton County, Ontario, of English parents who had come to Canada in pioneer days, doing their part in converting wilderness into fruitful fields. During 1854–5 he studied at Victoria University, intending to take a degree in Arts, but was forced to withdraw owing to ill health. In 1858 he entered the office of W. Case Adams of Toronto as a student of dentistry, and at the end of two years he began practising at the town of Milton, near his birthplace. He took an active interest in town affairs and soon held positions of trust, being appointed a Justice of the Peace and elected to the town council. In 1870–1 he attended the Philadelphia Dental College, graduating in 1871 at the head of his class with the degree of Doctor of Dental Surgery. In this same year he moved his dental office to Toronto. Throughout his life he was an ardent Liberal, thereby making friends and foes alike, but no one ever doubted his honesty. In religion, he was an active, devoted Methodist.

In 1868, the Ontario Dental Association had split into two organizations owing to disagreements. J.B. Willmott's first activity in organized dentistry was acting as secretary of a joint committee set up for a few months in 1869 to heal the breach. At an open meeting of licentiates in

1870, he was elected to the Ontario Board and a month later he was elected secretary of the Board, a position he held continuously until the time of his death in 1915.

Although he was a leader in all phases of Ontario dentistry for forty years, his greatest contribution was in the field of education. When the school opened in Toronto, the Board did not appoint a dean and for some strange reason actually did not establish the office, according to the official minutes, until 1893, when Willmott was appointed. From the beginning, however, he was head of the school. As such, he was not content to equal what was being done elsewhere, but strove to be ahead of others' efforts. Steadfastly he refused to compromise, and was stubborn in adhering to principle. He occupied the position of dean until the day of his death.

His son, Walter E. Willmott, graduated in 1888 and immediately came on the staff of the Toronto school, where he served in many capacities. On the death of his father, he succeeded as secretary of the Ontario Board. He served the profession in many capacities for over fifty years and was known as a personal friend to every Ontario dentist. Both father and son made great contributions to the progress of the profession during difficult times. For more than a half century, scarcely a page of the history of Ontario dentistry appears without the name of Willmott.

Luke Teskey earned his Licentiate in Dental Surgery by examination of the Ontario Board in 1873. Little is known respecting his personal history, but apparently he was practising dentistry and studying medicine when he was appointed with Willmott to establish the Toronto school in 1875. He graduated two years later from Trinity Medical College with the degree of Doctor of Medicine. Later he qualified with the Royal College of Surgeons in England and became a surgeon on the staff of the Toronto General Hospital. Teskey made a tremendous contribution to early dental education and served on the staff of the school for more than thirty years. From the beginning, he taught those subjects related to medicine. Latterly, his name appeared in the announcements as professor of principles and practice of medicine and surgery. He also served as registrar of the school for fifteen years. Between Willmott and Teskey the baselines of dental education were formulated.

The school opened in two rooms over a cabinet shop on 3 November 1875, with eleven students in attendance. The course lasted four months. During the two previous winters, Willmott had given evening lectures to indentured students preparing to take the licensure examination. A significant statement appeared in the first announcement of the school:

'While the Board have not, as yet, made attendance upon lectures a condition of examination, they now urge upon the students to attend at least one and if possible two courses. The licensure examinations in the future will be of such a character that it will be expedient for the student to avail himself of all possible assistance.'

At the time a student was required to be properly indentured with a qualified licentiate for two years before he could take the licensure examination. Nothing in the school's first announcement stated that students taking the course had to be indentured, nor was anything said respecting academic qualifications for admission to the course. During the first session, 120 patients were rendered gratuitous services in the infirmary; they came in greater numbers than could be attended by the students.

In their report to the Board following the close of the first session, Willmott and Teskey requested more space for the school. They also asked that all students thereafter articled should be required to attend two full courses of lectures in 'our own' school, and that the term of pupilage be shortened to two years, including the eight months spent attending lectures. The response to the latter request was contradictory in ruling and practice. The Board demanded that students be articled for three years and attend two full sessions in any reputable dental college before seeking admission to the licensure examination. However, the school's second announcement called only for a two year indenture, inclusive of the time spent in attendance upon lectures, before a student could sit for the licentiate. The annual grant was increased by $50 in order to provide more space. The number of professors was increased by the addition of Francis G. Callendar, C.S. Chittenden, H. Hipkins, and Thomas Rowe, but at the same time a motion was adopted permitting these men to discharge their duties by deputy – and that Messrs Willmott and Teskey be accepted as their deputies for this purpose. Presumably it was thought better to have additional names on the next announcement of the school even if the number of teachers was not materially increased. During the years that followed, the indentureship period was adjusted; the academic course was extended; a matriculation standard was set and altered from time to time; and as the number of students increased, the staff was enlarged and larger premises were secured for the school. It remained the only dental school in Canada until 1892.

By 1880, there were 351 registered dentists practising in Ontario and 117 in Quebec. The Atlantic provinces had no dental register as yet. The census for 1881 reported 510 dentists in the whole of Canada. In spite of law, there were men practising dentistry, or some phase of dentistry without a licence. Outside of Ontario and Quebec, it was difficult to determine who was truly entitled to be called a dentist, for little or no regulation existed.

A matter of concern was that, while extreme variation existed as to ability and skill among practitioners, there was no way of recognizing those with superior qualifications. As president of the Ontario Board, Henry T. Wood proposed application to the Legislature for amendment to the Dental Act to permit the creation of 'Fellows' of the Royal College of Dental Surgeons of Ontario.[9] The Legislature refused that change, but did amend the Act to permit the granting of the title, Master of Dental Surgery (MDS). To obtain the title, the candidate was required to pass an examination of high calibre and present a thesis. The Master's title became known as a degree, though the Board (as noted) had no right to confer degrees. The first title of Master of Dental Surgery was conferred in 1878 and the last in 1925, there being a total of 39. While few members in fact qualified, this action represented the first effective step towards higher academic standing.

In 1877, Hubbard's Dental Depot was advertising to dentists their stock of 'Crystal and corrugated Gold foils (Kearsing's, Valleau's, Pack's and Watt's); S.S. White's, Justi's and Johnson and Lund's Teeth, also cheap teeth for those who wish them; vulcanizers, forceps, pluggers, excavators, operating chairs, lathes, corrundum wheels, brushes, files, celluloid plates and all articles used by the profession.'[10] The advertisement made no mention of amalgam, which was freely in use. The 1870s' greatest innovation, which radically altered practice, was the introduction of the Morrison Dental Foot Engine. Up to this time hand instruments had been used entirely, and a good deal of scepticism arose at the introduction of a machine. J. A. Bazin, an outstanding dentist in Montreal, cited the dangers in 1878, the engine's worst feature in his eyes being 'that quantity removed at each revolution, as well as speed, engenders heat.'[11] He criticized the profession severely, on the grounds that ever since the introduction of the machine, 'so many minute fillings always in a nice place for a drill' were to be found in the mouths of patients. After castigating unscrupulous dentists, he raised a question that has been raised in years since in many forms: 'the engine is a convenient instrument, only in so far as it will, without doubt, do reliable work, or assist them to do the possible best for their patients; and it is to these I most earnestly press the question, has the public been and will it still be, the gainer by this machine?'

As previously stated, Charles A. Martin of Ottawa was a very popular after-dinner speaker in eastern Ontario for many years. He was perfectly bilingual, but usually apologized for his English when beginning an address. No meeting of the Eastern Ontario Dental Association (organized in 1880) was quite complete without an address by him. Having been a gunsmith in early life, he was an excellent mechanic. In one of his addresses, he related one of his experiences with a dental engine. He and his brother had laboured for several years in putting together pulleys and belts to operate a drill; then, just when they had the thing perfected, a Yankee pedlar came along with one ready to use. On another occasion he told in his inimitable manner the story of the best instrument in his cabinet. It had been made from a steel stay secured from his wife's corset! Unlike its original purpose, the use he had created for it promised to endure in perpetuity. The ingenuity of dentists of that time knew no bounds. They created instruments to suit their purposes, and in the process made the prototypes of instruments in use today.

Generally, it is observed, dentists up to the turn of the century were seized with the technical side of their profession. This is true, for if a health service was to be rendered at all, a great many technical problems had to be solved. There were many exceptions, however. At a meeting of the Dental Association of the Province of Quebec early in 1870, Pierre Baillargeon presented a dissertation on the effects of sugar upon the teeth. The lengthy discussion which followed had a modern ring. W.H. Patton of Montreal presented a forward approach to the subject of dental hygiene at the same time, and A.C. Stone of London stressed the importance of caring for children's teeth and the need for patient education. Other individual dentists were rising above the mechanics of dentistry; indeed, for years to come the main emphasis was on the education of the dentist. From the beginning of the Toronto school, the course laid weight on the basic sciences. Of two professors initially appointed, one had medical training. When a third professor was appointed in 1877, another medical doctor, W. Theophilis Stuart, was chosen. The need for a basic scientific emphasis is recognized today but the school was strongly criticized on this point for many years. The criticism was based on the old adage that philosophy bakes no bread.

In the newly created province of Manitoba, the population was still small. The earliest dentist of record to establish practice in Winnipeg was

James L. Benson. As a young man, he had gone west with the Wolsley expedition at the time of the Red River Rebellion in 1870, but had returned to his birthplace of Peterborough, Ontario, and then indentured with Jacob Neelands at Lindsay. In the latter 1870s, he moved west and established practice at Winnipeg, where he remained until his death in 1926.

The measure of a profession is sometimes assessed by the strength and development of its associations, schools, and journals. By the end of the seventies, the beginnings of each had occurred in Canadian dentistry. Associations of dentists existed in Quebec and Ontario, a school was in operation at Toronto, and the *Canada Journal of Dental Science* had been established. The organizations had gained varying strengths, but were dependent upon the efforts of a few dentists. The school at Toronto had made rather rapid progress since its establishment, and its future appeared assured. However, the *Journal* had faltered. George Beers was an excellent editor who realized the importance of a publication, but his effort was made as an individual and he exhausted his personal financial resources in attempting to provide a means of communication. The associations were neither ready nor in a position to give him the necessary support. Monthly issues of the *Journal* ended in May 1872. Then four issues followed during 1877 and 1878. The next decade passed without a journal, which seriously retarded the advancement of dentistry.

During this period Beers told the Quebec Dental Society: 'An infallible law exists with regard to all science and art, which, like that of the mutation of races and tongues, preserves the true or removes the imperfect, according to their development.'[12] To the leaders of dentistry, this was an exceedingly slow process, requiring abundant patience, time, and energy on the part of a few. For these years the dental literature contains many addresses on the same theme. C.P. Lennox, of Chatham pointed out to the Ontario Dental Society that education was the real basis of a profession, and not legislation as many dentists seemed to suppose. Further, he stated: 'It is a general conceived notion that the profession adds dignity to the man. This idea is false; it is the man who dignifies the profession.'[13] Statements made in many published addresses indicate deep concern respecting views, then currently expressed by dentists, which were considered detrimental to the future of dentistry as a profession.

6
Expansion
1880-1889

The opening of the West was the dominating feature of the 1880s. During the seventies, treaties had been signed with the various Indian tribes. The North West Mounted Police, later to become the Royal Canadian Mounted Police, had been formed to keep order in the vast territory. The land was surveyed, and with the completion of the Canadian Pacific Railway in November 1885 the area was ready for settlers. Many were attracted. Canada's first transcontinental passenger train left Montreal in June 1886 with several colonist cars full of hopeful and probably apprehensive homesteaders. In addition to this westward activity, eastern links were strengthened when the Intercolonial Railway between Haifax and Central Canada was completed in 1888.

The achievement of railway transportation from coast to coast initiated a period of rapid development in Canada as a whole. Cities grew from villages. Winnipeg became the commercial centre of the entire northwest and by 1890 had a population of over 25,000. Regina became the administrative centre for the territory and developed into a sizeable community of 2,000 persons. Calgary, which began as a North West Mounted Police fort erected at the junction of the Bow and Elbow rivers in 1875, consisted of only half a dozen log buildings when the Canadian Pacific Railway reached it in 1883, but by 1890 it had grown to nearly 4,000 people. Vancouver can be described as the city transportation built: before the CPR chose it as its western terminus, only a small lumbering village existed there; by 1891, its population was 13,700. With the completion of the Intercolonial Railway, Halifax gained in importance, becoming a city of 38,437 by 1891.

Dentistry followed the development of the country. Frederick Davis Shaw was the first established dentist in the whole of the North-West Territories, the enormous area which included all of what became the provinces of Alberta and Saskatchewan. Shaw was born at Kentville, Nova Scotia, of pioneer stock, the son of William Henry Shaw, MD, a prominent figure in that province. After attending Annapolis College, he obtained his degree as a veterinary surgeon. Later he graduated from a private dental school in the United States. He had difficulty, however, in establishing practice in his native province, and took a position as auditor with the Intercolonial Railway for four and a half years. But the call of the West was strong, and in 1880 he joined the North West Mounted Police. Shaw served in the force for four years, during which he was promoted to the rank of staff sergeant: his discharge certificate, dated 5 March 1884, states that he left in consequence of being invalided. At this time his father died, and he returned to Nova Scotia, married Agnes Madeline Moran of Halifax, and then moved her, together with his mother and family of three brothers, one sister and a nephew, to the West. They arrived in Calgary on one of the first Canadian Pacific trains in 1885, and then transferred to a stage coach for the final leg of the journey to Fort MacLeod, in what is now southern Alberta. The population of the area was scanty and scattered, but Shaw decided it was possible to open a dental practice. He applied to the North-West Territories Council at Regina for permission, which was granted. At the same time, he was granted permission to practise veterinary science. He provided himself with a buckboard and set up a regular schedule between Fort MacLeod, Pincher Creek, and Lethbridge. Shaw became an important citizen in the whole district. He was not only the first dentist and first veterinarian in the North-West Territories, but was also in time appointed Coroner and Collector of Customs in the St Mary's area. When the North-West Territories Dental Register was established in 1889, Shaw's name was the only one shown that year.

William Wilson, locally known as 'Tug' Wilson for obvious reasons related to his extractive services, was unquestionably the first dentist to practise at Calgary, though some confusion exists respecting the date.[1] In the city's first directory, published in 1885, he was the only dentist listed, together with an advertisement that he extracted teeth painlessly. Probably Wilson (a native of Kingston, Ontario) established practice at Calgary very soon after Shaw did so at MacLeod, but the question of which was first in the area may never be settled satisfactorily. At any rate, Shaw is first on the North-West Territories Register. Wilson's name appears the following year (1890), with Edmonton as his address. It may be that Wilson was wandering from place to place when Shaw established his practice. Both men had retired from the North West Mounted Police at about the same time. In 1966, John Clay, a prominent Calgary dentist, recalled that Wilson was practising there in a log shack near the junction of the Bow and Elbow rivers when he settled in Calgary in 1907.[2]

At Edmonton, the first dental practice was established by A.H. (Sandy) Goodwin in 1891, although the settlement had been visited by other dentists earlier. Goodwin was a native of Baie Verte, New Brunswick, and a member of the same family as W.S. Goodwin, who was later the first registered dentist in Newfoundland. He graduated from the Baltimore College of Dental Surgery in 1889 and after two years as a transient dentist in New Brunswick, left for the West. He arrived at his destination on the second train to run from Calgary to Edmonton, which then had a population of 1,500. The front parlour of Mrs. Kelly's log house on Jasper Avenue became his office at a rent of $10 a month.

Lorenzo D. Keown and his brother William set up practice at Regina in 1886. Theirs was said to be at the time the only dental practice between

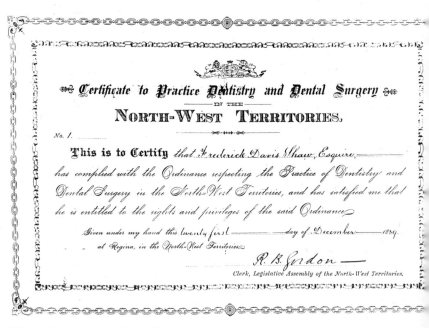

The first licence to practise dentistry in the North-West Territories

Brandon and Calgary, a distance of nearly 700 miles. Feeling that Regina had no future, Lorenzo moved to Moosomin, where he practised for over a half century. His brother remained in Regina, and died in 1899. Lorenzo Keown served on the Saskatchewan Dental Council for twenty-five years. His ability was recognized in many ways and he served in several public offices. In politics, he was a life-long Conservative and organized the party in the North-West Territories. In order to bring the benefits of his practice to the settlers, he made long trips by horse and buggy.

These men, and others who followed in bringing dentistry to the West, experienced many physical hardships, and had real problems earning a living from their practice alone. Establishing a dental office in town meant little as far as gaining a living was concerned. It was necessary to take dentistry to the scattered settlers, by any means available and over long distances. An even greater hindrance was the visitations of the travelling 'showman-type' dentist, who down-graded the profession in the eyes of the public. The following quotation describes Goodwin's opposition in Edmonton during the 1890s:[3]

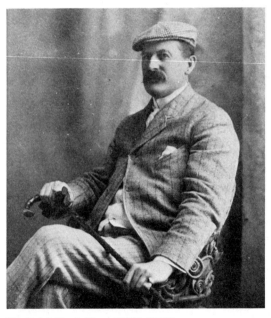

Frederick Davis Shaw (1856–1926)

His only competition came from a travelling charlatan – the amazing, the incredible 'Dr' True. 'Dr' True used to hit town twice a year, travelling with two ladies, a drum, and a set of tongs. 'Dr' True was late-thirtyish, with a Buffalo Bill haircut, a pale face, piercing eyes and an even more piercing voice. He would ride up and down Jasper, beating the drum, until he drew a crowd. Then he'd exhibit a basket of bills, and for five dollars you could stick your hand in and take a chance on pulling out a ten-dollar bill or a twenty, or a one. Then he'd sell charms – charms that would ward off anything, including pain. If you bought a charm the amazing 'Dr' True would yank one of your teeth – right there in the dust of Jasper Avenue – to prove that the charm warded off pain. He used the same tongs for every tooth and between extractions would clean them off on his trousers. People who bought charms wouldn't care to admit they'd been taken in, so they would testify that the yanking didn't hurt a bit. Dr Goodwin got some business out of the amazing 'Dr' True's dentistry – treating the infections and fishing out the roots.

Following the achievements in Ontario and Quebec during the late 1860s, dentists in Canada's other provinces endeavoured to obtain legislative recognition. An Act establishing the Manitoba Dental Association was passed in 1883, mainly as a result of the efforts of James L. Benson, referred to in the last chapter, who became the first president. In British Columbia, the chief protagonist was Thomas J. Jones, who was born in Toronto, began studying dentistry in 1860, and practised in Bowmanville and St. Catharines for twenty years, during which period he served as president of the Ontario Dental Society. In 1884, he moved to Victoria, where he practised for another forty years. Coming from Ontario where a dental act existed, he very naturally agitated for legislation in British Columbia, and succeeded in 1886. During the following three years, twenty-one persons were licensed to practise dentistry in the province, eleven of them in Victoria, four in Vancouver, four in New Westminster, and one each in Nanaimo and Barkerville. One of them possessed a degree both in medicine and dentistry, nine had doctoral degrees in dentistry, and three had obtained licentiate standing (LDS) elsewhere.[4] Apparently an informal provincial dental society existed earlier but the British Columbia Dental Association was not founded until 1891. At its first annual meeting in Victoria, in 1891, Jones (its principal organizer) was elected president. In a special edition of the Victoria *Daily Colonist* in April 1896, Thomas Jones was credited with being a foremost citizen: in addition to his large modern practice, it reported, he had various other

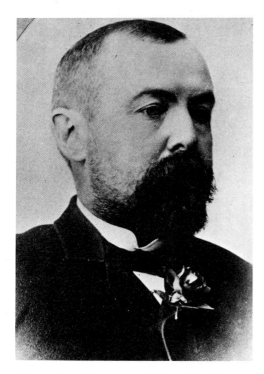

Thomas Joseph Jones, LDS, father of dentistry in
British Columbia

interests and was considered an enterprising, public-spirited citizen. His
activities on behalf of the profession entitle him to recognition as Father
of Dentistry in British Columbia.

New Brunswick obtained legislation in 1890, and in both Nova Scotia
and Prince Edward Island dental acts were enacted by the respective legislatures during 1891. Legislation came about in Newfoundland in 1893.
The North-West Territories Council adopted an Ordinance for the control
of dental practice in 1889 – but without consulting dentists and it was only
as a result of amendments secured by W.D. Cowan of Regina that it
became a workable measure. Legislation followed more normal routes on
the Atlantic coast. In each province, some one dentist was responsible
for first gaining the support of his colleagues for the objectives of a dental
act, and then having the patience and endurance necessary to secure the

legislation. History does not produce men; it is men who make history. In New Brunswick, after others had failed, C.A. Murray of Moncton was successful. The Act he fought for established the New Brunswick Dental Society with powers similar to those granted its counterparts in other provinces. A.J. McAvenney of Saint John was the first president.

Alfred Chipman Cogswell, a member of one of Nova Scotia's most prominent families, was the province's leading dentist from the 1860s to the turn of the century.[5] Born in Cornwallis, NS, in 1834, he attended Acadia College for two years, spent a couple of years on his father's farm near Portland, Maine, and then indentured with Edwin Parsons of that city. He practised a few years in New England and in 1859 moved to Halifax. He attended Philadelphia Dental College during one winter, graduating in 1869. That same year, following the enactment of legislation in Ontario, he made his first attempt to secure legislation in Nova

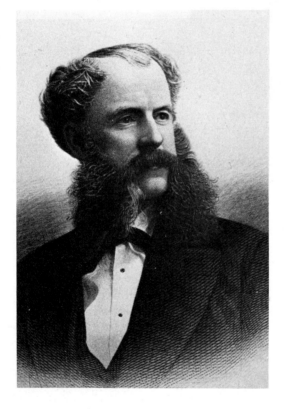

Alfred Chipman Cogswell, DDS, of Halifax (1834–1904)

Scotia. This effort failed, owing to the de Cheverie affair related earlier. For twenty years he pursued the objective. During this period, practically all the information respecting dentistry in Nova Scotia that appeared in the dental literature came from his pen. It is said of him that no one man worked more incessantly for so many years endeavouring to elevate his profession. He was instrumental in bringing about the Act which finally incorporated the Nova Scotia Dental Association in 1891. Cogswell was a great traveller and in 1904, on one of his many trips, he was accidentally shot in Mexico City.

During 1891, as in Nova Scotia, a dental Act came into force in Prince Edward Island, though it did not name an association or society as governing body. Doubtless, this difference from legislation in the other provinces occurred because of the small number of dentists – only seven then practising on the island could qualify. The Act was secured through the efforts of one man, John S. Bagnall, father of J. Stanley Bagnall, who became dean at Dalhousie University. It was not until 1901 that an association was formed, with the elder Bagnall its first president. Later, through amendment to the Act, the association was made the governing body of the profession.

In 1893, the Colonial Government in Newfoundland enacted a dental Act, thus completing legislation for dentistry across the whole country. Since then these original dental acts have been amended on many occasions, but the principle of self-governing professions has been adhered to. This achievement represented a great deal of arduous, often discouraging, struggle by a few dentists in each province. Today the accomplishment is taken for granted, but for more than twenty years recognition by legislatures was a prime professional objective.

Probably one of the most notable events in the development of the dental profession occurred in 1888 when the dental school at Toronto was affiliated with the University of Toronto. The university established a Department of Dentistry (Royal College of Dental Surgeons) and agreed to confer the degree of Doctor of Dental Surgery upon students on compliance with the requirements of the curriculum in dentistry as approved by the University Senate. In essence, under the agreement future matriculation standards, curricula, and examinations were to have the approval of the university. The first examination for the degree occurred in March 1889, when twenty-five candidates were successful. These were the first doctorate degrees conferred on dental graduates outside of the United States.

Next to the incorporation of dentistry in Ontario (1868) and the establishment of a dental school (1875), this affiliation represented the greatest move forward by the profession to that date. The academic standing of dentists was elevated. While several men made periodic contributions towards the goal, J.B. Willmott worked continuously for it for some twenty years, and in reality deserves credit for its attainment. On the university side, William (later Sir William) Mulock, vice-chancellor at the time, persuaded his colleagues to recognize dentistry. By this time, Willmott had become an outstanding citizen, known for his service to dentistry as well as public affairs. In the next announcement of the school, J.B. Willmott was shown as dean for the first time. [6]

In tracing the development of the profession, the impression must not be left that gains were achieved in logical sequences or easily. Perhaps the greatest handicap came from dentists themselves. Criticism of leaders and their objectives was severe and at times malicious, illustrating ignorance or lack of understanding. One illustration, a letter received from a dentist and the reply from George Beers as editor of the *Journal*, will suffice to exemplify a state of affairs which was altogether too prevalent.[7] The letter Beers received read:

I am not a subscriber to the Journal, and I don't mean to be, and I'll give you my reasons: You take too high a stand to start with, as the profession is new in Canada, and the dentists cannot afford to starve for the sake of keeping up appearances, societies and journals. I never asked anybody for ideas, and I don't give any. I do not trouble anyone. If you choose to crack up education, I will not quarrell with you. Only I have so far satisfied a good majority of the people for over twenty-eight years or more, and I think my work will speak for itself. I would not have ninety-nine out of every one hundred of your 'educated' young men in my office. They think they know so much; you discover they know very little, though they can talk theory to you, and have more brag, and gas than real ability. Just let dentistry slip along in the old way, and if you have any practical hints give them to us and we can pay for them. But I say we don't want 'highly-educated' men. We want good mechanics, who can work in their shirt sleeves, and who aren't particular about all the fine nonsense of antiseptics, bacteria etc. What the mischief does it all mean? Am I a fool, or are you.

Beers replied in an editorial:

If the kicker had his way in Canada, instead of organized means of education, we should find stable boys and jewellers jumping from the curry-comb and the bench into the surgery at one bound, after perhaps six weeks training. The kicker, as a rule, who condemns education because it is not equal to the very best order and more populous countries supply, is well aware that he himself is unqualified to improve it, and the impracticable suggestions he ever ventures to make only prove that he is more animated by jealousy and ignorance than any idea of self-sacrifice or sincerity. He is as lavish in unreasonable criticism as he is niggardly of his time or money ... The kicker has rarely, if ever, distinguished himself by self-sacrifice.

Advertising in every possible form became the most serious impediment to those endeavouring to elevate the profession. In the language of the day, offenders were conducting 'quackish' practices by means of 'claptrap' advertisements and 'cheap John' performances. The public suffered the consequences. By 1887, 8 × 12 foot boards stood at every public road entrance to the city of Toronto, setting forth in fourteen-inch-high letters the names and addresses of dentists who emphasized cheapness and nothing more. Evidence of the horrible extremities reached are to be found in old newspapers, handbills, and cards. Advertising by dentists seemed to reach a crescendo by the turn of the century; after that it diminished, slowly and over several decades. Amendments to dental laws and reform movements initiated within dental organizations finally brought advertising under control, but all this took a distressingly long time.

Both in Quebec and Ontario, the dental boards fought the issue with all the tools at their command. The records of the voluntary societies are filled with discussions as to methods to counter the advertiser. At one point the Ontario Dental Society fell under the control of the advertisers, and for a few years little record of its activities has survived. In 1889, however, a group of ethical dentists called a meeting at London, and with forty-six members in attendance made every effort to dissociate from the former society. The objectives of the society were altered, and with considerable emphasis that meeting was numbered One. The main business was the adoption of a code of ethics which strictly prohibited advertising. To become a member of the new society, each applicant had to sign this code. Nearly all the dentists present signed. Although advertising continued, even increasing somewhat after this date, the Ontario meeting represented a turning point. In proof it is tempting to include at considerable length details of a battle which took place within the profession over far too many years, and greatly hindered its development. Many dentists were involved, in increasing numbers, against the cancer of advertising, chiefly under the leadership of Beers in Quebec and Willmott in Ontario.

The foundation of dentistry was greatly strengthened by a journalistic revival. The *Dominion Dental Journal* was established, the first issue appearing in January 1889 with W. George Beers as editor. An amicable arrangement had been made whereby the faltered *Canada Journal of Dental Science* was taken over by the new publication. For the first year, this new journal was issued quarterly; in the second year it became bi-monthly, and in 1893 monthly. It was published in Toronto and served the profession well over forty years, when it was absorbed by the *Journal of the Canadian Dental Association*. From this time forward, dentists in Canada possessed a means of communication which had been sadly lacking for seventeen years. The need of a profession for adequate means of intercourse can hardly be better illustrated than by the vacant interval. In covering this period, the historian is left with only scanty records, public archives, old newspapers, and extraneous publications as sources of information.

The economics of the times are illustrated in an account for services rendered by G.E. Hanna, who later became president of the Ontario Board. Hanna represents well the practising dentist of the period. The account form not only lists the services rendered and fees charged, but also contains a fee schedule. The services were rendered for a family of three children. Miss Lizzie had nine fillings performed for five dollars, Miss Maggie's tooth was extracted for twenty-five cents, while Angus cost his parents a dollar for one filling and an extraction. The total account for the three amounted to $13.75, but two gallons of maple syrup and two cords of wood at a dollar a cord are credited. Barter items were common on many dental accounts. Orthodontists might note that the fee for correcting irregularities of teeth varied all the way from two to ten dollars. Other accounts examined for the 1880s are comparable.

Charles Nelson Johnson was born in a farming community in Ontario and graduated from the Royal College of Dental Surgeons in 1881. He established practice at Collingwood and while there published a pamphlet entitled, *The Teeth, their Importance and How to Preserve Them*, which had wide circulation. At the end of three years, he went to Chicago where he became one of the most outstanding American dentists, occupying the highest positions the profession had to offer. Yet even while living in Chi-

FEES.

FILLING.

With Gold (Simple)..... $1 to $3
" (Compound).. 2 to 5
Amalgam (Silver) .... 50c to $1
Porcelain Cement ...... 75c & up
Other Cements ...... 50c "
Removing Nerve and
Filling Root. .... 75c to $1

MECHANICAL.

Full Sets plain teeth, on
Rubber .... $10 to 12
Gum Teeth, on Rubber. 12 to 18
Plain Teeth, on Celleloid 12 to 15
Gum " " ...... 15 to 18
On Solid Gold Plate. .. 30 to 50
On Solid Silver " .. 25 to 30
Partial Sets from $3 upwards.

☞ TERMS CASH.

MALEY BLOCK.

Kemptville *July 19th,* 1881

Mr. Alex. Buchanan

G. E. HANNA, L.D.S.,

SURGEON DENTIST.

FEES.

SURGICAL.

Extracting Teeth ......25 to 50c.
Nerve treatment ......25 to 50c.
Operation on Abscess ......25c.
Correcting irregularities
of Teeth .... $2 to $10
N. O. Gas, each exhibition $1.50
Chloroform or Ether
each exhibition $1 00

NOTE— All operations not paid for when completed will be charged extra; also extra charges will be made for operations done before or after hours and on Sundays.

A typical account of the 1880s

cago, he made a great contribution to Canadian dentistry. Over a period of forty years, his name appeared on the convention programs of the Ontario Dental Association more often than that of any other person.[8] He was a prolific writer, and contributed generously to Canadian dental literature articles that were read with avid interest. The University of Toronto honoured him in 1932 with the degree of Doctor of Laws. Seldom has a man, spending his life in another country, done so much for his profession in his native land. At his death in 1938, Canadian dentistry paid him glowing tribute. Earlier, at a luncheon given in his honour at Toronto in 1924, it was said of him: 'He helped his fellow men,' and 'He stooped to aid a fallen comrade whenever he saw one down and put a prop under those whom he found trembling in the balance.'[9]

Coming-of-age celebrations in the central provinces occurred in 1889, when progress to date was assessed and predictions made for the future. C.F.F. Trestler, president of the Quebec Board, pointed out that in comparison with Ontario his province faced two main difficulties – numerical weakness in the ranks of the profession and dual languages – that made progressive activities costly. Owing to lack of support for dental services, it was not yet considered practicable to establish a dental school in Quebec. French students were in the majority and existing dental schools taught in English only; but public demand would not warrant the establishment of two teaching bodies. One of the great difficulties in Quebec was to deal effectively with quacks and unlicensed practitioners. However, amendments to the dental law had just been obtained which, it was said, would handle this matter with efficiency. Trestler was one of the founders of dentistry in Quebec. He was a medical graduate, and one of the earliest dentists in Canada to use chloroform and nitrous oxide in his practice.

In Ontario, the recent affiliation of the dental school with the University of Toronto was the main achievement put forth at anniversary meetings. A tendency existed to consider professional maturity attained, but J.B. Willmott warned in stern language that dentists had not yet cultivated in themselves that respect and enthusiasm for their profession that would engender respect from the public. He noted the absence of such professional etiquette as would indicate full professional maturity: dentists were too much disposed to misrepresent and take advantage of one another through advertising. Dentistry had made giant strides forward, but further advancement depended upon correcting situations which existed within the profession. It was also noted with surprise that after the long struggle for affiliation, a second Ontario university had, without knowledge or behest of the profession, given notice of the introduction of a statute to establish a curriculum in dentistry leading to a degree.

The twenty-first birthday was a time of review, when the founders and principal contributors to advancement were honoured. In Quebec, the names of Bernard, Baillargeon, Trestler, Brewster, LeBlanc, Beers, Bazin, and Webster were placed in the hall of dental fame. In Ontario, the names of men like Day, Wood, Relyea, Chittenden, O'Donnell, and Willmott were referred to with pride. Unfortunately, time had taken its toll among the early stalwarts, C.S. Chittenden, an energetic worker in every good effort, died during this year. Day and Relyea had gone to United States, and O'Donnell had died in 1879. In Quebec, Bernard died in 1876. Baillargeon was to die a year later, Webster had died, and Brewster had retired. LeBlanc carried on as secretary for six years more. Beers and Willmott now were the outstanding men of dentistry in the two provinces. Fortunately, other hands, in increasing numbers, had come forward to replace those who had gone, and were carrying on the work.

The wide range of activities of W. George Beers and his lasting influence on Canadian life are remarkable. He was an intense patriot and in demand as a public speaker. In 1888, at a time of political disturbances between the United States and Canada, he addressed the New York State Dental Society at Syracuse on the subject, 'Canada Not For Sale.' His words were terse and undoubtedly the audience were surprised to hear him say: 'I am sure that you could have nothing but contempt for any free people who measure their allegiance purely by commercial standards, and who, fearing to face the difficulties which meet every nation, turn peddlers instead of protectors of their national birthright. Just as you had and have your croakers and cowards we have ours, but Mr Chairman, Canada is not for sale.' This event would mean little if it were not for the aftermath. Canadian newspapers printed the speech widely, and for many years after, editorials referred to it. The address was an influential factor in the federal election in 1911, when it was used freely, and as late as 1916, some sixteen years after his death, it was reprinted in full. Few members of the dental profession have attained his public stature.

Among the names which appeared during these years, that of James Wellington Ivory became familiar to every practising dentist. He was born at Newcastle, Ontario, graduated from the Royal College of Dental Surgeons in 1887, and practised in Toronto for six years. His hobby was inventive mechanics. Leaving Toronto, he went to Philadelphia, where he established the firm of J.W. Ivory, Inc, specializing in the manufacture of dental instruments. During his lifetime, he held a great number of patents and his instruments were readily accepted.[10]

By 1889, there were 21 dentists registered in British Columbia, 40 in Nova Scotia, 117 in Quebec, and 494 in Ontario. The other provinces had only few dentists. By modern standards, these numbers represented a poor service for a country of five million people. Even in Ontario, the largest province, the ratio was less than one dentist for four thousand of the population. Lack of public appreciation for dental services was a great problem which would be the target of an increasing effort on the part of all dental organizations.

Always, change comes hard to some, and often most hard for those who have achieved the most under the old system. During this period Oliver Martin commented: 'We had a trade with principles, and now have a profession with none.' Some truth existed for his statement. Dentists were going through a transition period and it took some time to adapt themselves to a new environment. The principles of a trade were well understood; the ethics of a profession had yet to be learned.

7
Technical advancement
1890-1899

During the hiatus in the progress of the Ontario Dental Society referred to in the preceding chapter, the Eastern Ontario Dental Association became actively engaged in the affairs of the profession, mainly under the inspiration of Charles A. Martin of Ottawa. Insidious rumours, initially discussed at EODA meetings, spread among Ontario dentists that the professors at the Toronto school were becoming rich out of the profits from the school. At the 1890 annual meeting of the rejuvenated Ontario Dental Society, President G.C. Davies emphatically stated 'that the Dental College should be managed by the Board of Directors of the Royal College of Dental Surgeons of Ontario, that all fees should be paid to the Board, they to assume its liabilities.[1]

When the school was founded in 1875, the Ontario Board had very carefully placed the financial responsibility for its operation on the shoulders of the two appointed professors, Willmott and Teskey. The Board had made certain, as far as possible, that it would have no responsibility for any deficit, such as had developed with the abortive school of 1869. It voted only a small grant of $400 to cover rent and furnishings. Willmott and Teskey operated the school out of the student fees, and if any money was left at the end of the year, the staff was paid on a pro-rata basis. The Board however retained control through the appointment of staff, the setting of matriculation standards, the setting of the number of sessions, the amount of the academic fee, and the curriculum content. By the 1888–9 session, the number of students in attendance had increased to fifty. Finances related to the school were kept entirely separate from

those of the Board, and at no time do the records show a financial statement on the operation of the school. At meetings, the dissident dentists
argued that the Board should take over complete operation of the school,
issue full financial statements, and pay salaries to the staff. Between
meetings, exaggerated rumours were rife and the whole matter became
one of heated controversy for two or three years. The principles involved
were right, but the details discussed were incorrect. Over the years, the
professors, as they were termed (sometimes with derision during heated
arguments), had received very little recompense; some years nothing at
all was left for division. Undoubtedly they had made a mistake in
not issuing annual financial statements, but no such request had been
made. In fact, recorded discussions suggest that all financial aspects had
been avoided by the Board, who were content to let Willmott and Teskey
bear the responsibility. Even with the school established, the Board found
the position somewhat awkward. The matriculation standard, now a university matter, was being raised, and a reduction in the number of students
was anticipated. After lengthy discussions, however, the Board finally
accepted financial control. To modern eyes, perhaps, the magnitude of the
whole argument is somewhat diminished with the statement that the salary
of the dean was set in 1893 at $250 per year.

A good deal of rivalry existed among educational institutions during
this period. After the years of effort spent by the Ontario Board in securing an affiliation agreement with the University of Toronto, the formation
of a dental faculty at the University of Trinity College (to give that
institution its full and proper name) was a considerable surprise. The
records of the Royal College of Dental Surgeons of Ontario do not indicate any consultation or agreement with Trinity. In fact, almost the only
mention found of that university in Ontario dental records is its conferring
of an honorary doctorate in 1903 on G.E. Hanna, a former president of
the Ontario Board. The first doctorate in dentistry conferred by Trinity
College was upon Albert W. Spaulding in 1890.

The calendars issued by the Dental Faculty of Trinity College
state that graduates from any recognized university or the Royal College
of Dental Surgeons would be recognized for examination. It is interesting
to note that, at the beginning, the staff listed consisted of W.T. Stuart and
Luke Teskey, who also served on the staff of the Royal College of Dental
Surgeons, together with C.A. Snelgrove, F.J. Capon, and C. Sheard, who
were prominent Toronto dentists. At a later date J.B. Willmott, A.E.
Webster, and R.J. Reade joined the Trinity staff – which was larger in the

calendar lists than that of the Royal College of Dental Surgeons. Difficulty is found, however, in finding evidence of actual lectures or clinical training of any kind being given by Trinity. It appears that the staff acted as examiners for the degree of Doctor of Dental Surgery. In total, some sixty-six degrees were conferred by Trinity in dentistry, five of them honorary. The last holder of a Trinity degree, Oliver A. Marshall of Belleville, died in 1957. During 1903, Trinity and the University of Toronto joined in federation, and under the agreement, Trinity gave up all degree-conferring powers except in divinity. No further degrees in dentistry or medicine were conferred. The University of Toronto recognized those which had been conferred by Trinity.[2]

Progress in the development of dental services cannot be judged solely by official actions taken, for often it took many years to bring the intent of such actions to fruition. In the major centres of population, it is true, dental services were by this time receiving increasing recognition, but large rural areas existed where little improvement was noticeable. In spite of legislative authority, the dental boards found control of quacks difficult. I spent my early childhood in one of the poorer areas, and can remember that as late as 1904 it was a debatable point among the populace whether it was better to have a local farmer extract an aching tooth with his turnkey or drive six miles to a dentist with his cruel forceps. The education of the public to professional dental services was a slow process.

To obtain a perspective on the manner of change, it may be well to follow the career of a single dentist. John N. Brimacombe practised at Bowmanville, Ontario, from the early 1860s until his death in 1908. In 1899 he was elected president of the Ontario Dental Society. When he died, the local newspaper described him a very esteemed citizen who wrote his name in kindness, love, and mercy on the hearts of those whom he met from day to day, and said that many a poor and needy family had been made richer or better by his gifts.[3] His life story illustrates the changed position of the dentist over a period of half a century in a relatively small community.

Like many other young men, Brimacombe arrived in the Bowmanville area from England during the early 1850s. In a few years he had saved $400, a considerable sum in those days, from working at several occupations. He became interested in dentistry, and was referred to a Toronto dentist, W. Case Adams. But two years' indentureship with Adams at a fee of $200 was more than his pocketbook could stand, so he signed indenture papers for eighteen months at a fee of $100 with an Oshawa dentist named Vars. His preceptor's library was small: it consisted of only two books – Goddard's *The Anatomy, Physiology, and Pathology of the Human Teeth* and Harris' *Principles and Practises of Dentistry*. An incident during his indentureship is best told by Brimacombe himself:[4]

> But the worst piece of downright cheek was when my preceptor sent me (armed with turnkey) many miles into the country to extract a lower wisdom tooth for a lady still in bed recovering after confinement. Operation performed on my knees. Strange to say it was considered a great success, and after forty-two years she still enjoys good health. Being of a charitable disposition, she considers herself fortunate to be numbered amongst my patients, as well as her children and grandchildren. Wishing to retain her friendship, I took the advice of *Punch's Almanac*, which says some things ought never to be told.

When Brimacombe set up his practice in Bowmanville, it was not possible to make a living in a small community from dentistry alone; being musical, he became an agent for a piano company to supplement his income. Later he was appointed telegraph agent, a position he held for several years. He was an able dentist for his time, but it was not until the late 1880s that he could afford to confine his activities to his practice. Most dentists had similar experiences up to the 1890s, and even beyond this period.

Due to the spatial nature of Canada, experiences were repeated as each area opened up for settlement over a long span of years. Medical graduates for many years found forceps an essential part of their equipment. The story is vividly told of Murrough O'Brien, an early graduate (in 1897) of the Manitoba Medical College at Winnipeg.[5] He established practice in southern Manitoba at Dominion City, a village with a big sounding name. His first patients were for tooth extractions, and his reputation was established by his proficiency in that operation. In newly settled areas, a mechanic or farmer often established a similar reputation for extracting teeth, albeit in a cruder fashion. Toothache was not constrained to await the arrival of a qualified practitioner.

In 1896, S.W. McInnis of Brandon, Manitoba, published an article describing his country practice. 'The patients of the city, whether resident or visiting, are educated to a great extent as to the value of their teeth and the possibilities of dentistry. With people living in villages and the outlying country it is not so, at least not so much so. The farmers' creed is very simple – "if your tooth aches have it pulled." The brushing and cleansing of teeth are to the ordinary farmer like wearing a white shirt, an uncalled for and snobbish extravagance. The farmer's wife or daughter looks forward to the time when she can have as pretty a new set of teeth as her neighbour, with a longing proportionate to the envy, ambition and vanity of her nature. This ignorance, this lack of education, is one of the foremost difficulties to be encountered in a country practice.' He went on to describe his practice, which involved visits to several villages within a radius of fifty miles of his house ('my head office'). He said that patients presented their mouths with teeth in all stages of irregularity, decay, and disease. They were not rich, did not value their teeth, and were not willing to spend much time or money on them.[6]

During this period, Quebec, under the twin handicaps of two languages and few dentists, struggled toward the establishment of a school. After a great deal of negotiation, the Dental College of the Province of Quebec opened courses at Montreal in the fall of 1892, with W. George Beers as dean. Instruction was given in both French and English, with lectures in medical subjects taken at McGill and Laval Universities.[7] The Dental Board leased a building on Phillips Square, Montreal, for the

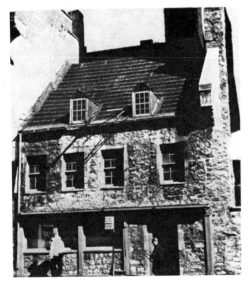

Home of Quebec's first dental school, the Dental College of the Province of Quebec, at 2 Phillips Square, Montreal

school, and made a grant of $500 toward equipment. The course was three years in length, one year more than the indentureship period in Quebec at the time.

After a successful first year of operation, the Dental Board sought university affiliation for the school so that graduates would receive the degree of Doctor of Dental Surgery. Letters making the request were sent to both Laval and McGill. For some reason, not very clear, Laval could not accept the overture for affiliation. McGill was willing to accept the proposal conditionally by granting a degree of Graduate of Dental Surgery (GDS) which the Dental Board found meaningless and unacceptable. There was, however, a third medical school in Montreal, operated by the University of Bishop's College, Lennoxville, from 1871 to 1905, when it was merged with the Medical Faculty of McGill. The fact that Bishop's had been ignored by the Dental Board resulted in some dispute, but eventually a compromise was reached. In 1896, a Department of Dentistry was formed in Bishop's Faculty of Medicine by affiliation of the Quebec Dental College. Teaching was in both French and English. Bishop's thus became the first university in Quebec to provide a dental course leading to the degree of Doctor of Dental Surgery.

An event occurred in the same province during 1896 which influenced the attitude of the profession in respect to the employment of auxiliary personnel in dental offices for many years in future. In order to understand its import, it is necessary to summarize the indentureship arrangement at that time. In all provinces, indentureship with a registered dentist was originally the only form of training. When dental education became available, attendance at the sessions of a school really became a part of the indentureship term. The student still had to sign an indenture contract with a registered dentist for a stated term of years, and during those years he was required to attend sessions of the school in order to qualify for the licensure examination. Of course, abuses of the system occurred. Some contracts were broken by students who attempted to practise illegally, and some dentists took advantage of the students by using them for their own profit rather than training them. The important point in this context is that no person except a registered dental student was permitted to work with a licensed dentist in a dental office.

A group of Quebec dentists, however, without consultation with the Dental Board, submitted a petition in 1896 to the Quebec Legislature, requesting an amendment to the Dental Act to permit the employment of dental assistants. Several members of the staff of the dental school signed the petition, and as a result George Beers resigned as dean. A general uproar ensued. The Dental Board circularized the profession, pointing out that the requested amendment would make a licence to practise unnecessary, that the door would be opened to the extension of branch offices conducted by such assistants, and that a class of practitioners would be established who would seriously injure qualified dentists and registered students. A second petition was forwarded to the legislature, signed by most dentists who had signed the first one, requesting withdrawal of their names. As a result no action was taken. Beers, however, refused to withdraw his resignation, which was finally accepted with regret and with gratitude for all he had accomplished for dentistry. Stephen Globensky was appointed his successor. Globensky had been one of the most active dentists in organizing the profession in Quebec. His great-grandfather was listed under the *saigneurs et aracheurs de dents* of the French regime, and he himself had served many years on the Quebec Board and had been a member of the staff of the school from the beginning.

The first Canadian woman to graduate from a dental school was Mrs. C.L. Josephine Wells, who completed the course at the Royal College of

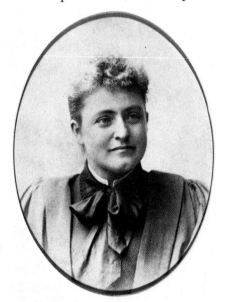

Caroline Louisa Josephine Wells,
first woman graduate in dentistry in Canada

Dental Surgeons in 1893.[8] Later, encouraged by her friends, she took the examination at Trinity College and obtained her doctorate in 1899. Her husband, John Wells, had graduated in dentistry in 1882 as gold medallist of his year, and when his health became poor, she decided to follow his profession. She practised most creditably for some thirty-six years, during which she became very interested in institutional dentistry. She is credited with initiating dental services in Ontario Mental Hospitals, and confined herself entirely to practice in those hospitals for ten years before her retirement. She died in 1939 in her 83rd year. Of her five children, the youngest, the Honourable Dalton C. Wells, was appointed Chief Justice of the High Court of Ontario in 1966. I acted as assistant to Dr Wells at the Toronto Mental Hospital during one winter and can vouch for her intelligent approach to dental treatment for mental patients.

Annie Grant Hill was the first woman to be granted a licence to practise in Quebec by examination, in 1893.[9] She practised for a time in Montreal but little is known of her except that she married and had left that province by 1899. The story of Madame Emma Casgrain, who was the second woman to practise in Quebec, is well recorded. She was granted a licence *pro forma* in 1898. Her husband, H. Edmond Casgrain,

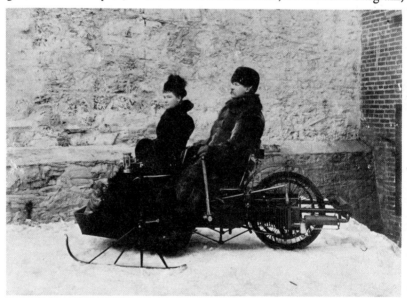

H.E. Casgrain and Mme Casgrain of Quebec in the first snowmobile, which he invented

who was also a dentist, served on the Quebec Board for several years and took considerable interest in public affairs. He was moreover an artist and inventor of some magnitude and held a sizeable number of patents. He is credited as the first Canadian to own a motor car – one with three wheels which he bought in France in February 1897. Among his inventions is listed the first snowmobile (1898), which was described in an article in the *Scientific American* for that year.[10] He has also been described as a great sportsman. Probably all these activities of her husband were factors in Madame Casgrain's decision to practise dentistry; she may also have been influenced by the example of her brother, Stanislas Gaudreau, a successful dentist in Quebec City for many years. (A nephew, Gustave Ratte, was president of the Canadian Dental Association in 1952–3.) Mrs Wells, Miss Hill and Madame Casgrain were the pioneer women in Canadian dentistry, and no others appeared for some years.

The 1890s were a period of considerable technical advance on many fronts. There was great interest, for example, in any new drug which became available. Many were introduced into dental practice, received enthusiastic support for a short period, and later discarded. Endorsement was based usually upon clinical experience rather than scientific proof. In an address to the Ontario Dental Society on the subject in 1892, W.E. Willmott presented three drugs recently introduced in dental practice which were then considered valuable. Aristol (dithymol-biniodide) was stated to be non-irritating, non-poisonous, and while similar to iodoform in use did not have its disgusting odour or its toxic properties. Hydrogen peroxide, discovered in 1818, was just coming into surgical use. Camphophenique was comparatively new, and advocated for use as an antiseptic.

Three techniques for treatment came into vogue during the 1890s at least two of which seem to possess great powers of recurrence at intervals. The first was mesmerism, or hypnosis as it became named, which was introduced in Europe by Franz Mesmer, an Austrian mystic and physician, during the middle years of the eighteenth century. He was called an imposter and a charlatan by physicians of the time. A paper presented by a famous professor from Harvard University at the 1896 annual meeting of the Ontario Dental Society initiated a revival of its use in Canadian dental practice. Since then the subject has reappeared in dental programs at fairly regular intervals of ten to fifteen years, receiving perhaps its greatest attention in Canada during the mid-1900s.

Implantation of teeth has also had its vogues ever since John Hunter

(1728–93) carried out the first experiments in England, based upon his belief in a natural tendency of all vital tissues to unite when closely approximated. The original preserved experiment of implanting a tooth in a cock's comb, when observed in the Hunterian Collection of the Royal College of Surgeons of England, still is fascinating. Following Hunter, various dentists attempted it, but seldom with success; later Hunter himself stated that, out of a great number of trials, he had succeeded but once.[11] A revival of interest in implantation occurred in Canada during the 1890s, when J.B. Willmott reported apparent success at a meeting of the Ontario Dental Society. Considerable further research took place on this continent during the mid-1900s, without much practical result in general practice. From time to time, the subject has re-appeared in Canadian dental literature.

Following the introduction of electricity in dental practice came the third prominent technique introduced during this period, cataphoresis. This was a method of introducing medicine into the system by means of an electric current. Dentists used it for root canal treatment. For several years, a convention program was hardly complete without a paper on this subject. Its value for treatment was greatly enhanced by prominent speakers, and enthusiasm for its use continued for several years before adequate research established that it was not in fact beneficial. In the meantime, elaborate equipment for cataphoric treatment appeared on the market. As late as the 1920s such equipment was to be found in modern dental offices, although by that time its usefulness had been discounted.[12]

Numerous other developments occurred during this period which did have lasting value. Electricity was coming into general use and was to cause the second great alteration in dental practice, the introduction of vulcanite having been the first. Strange to say, while the first electric engine with a flexible shaft had been invented in 1883, it was cataphoresis which first caught the imagination of dentists, at least judging by papers presented at their meetings.

One of the key figures in the electrical revolution was Frank DeMille Price, a Toronto dentist from 1892 to 1935. He was the type of man who fascinates the student of history. One of a family of twelve, he was born on a farm near Napanee, Ontario, in 1866, graduated from the Royal College of Dental Surgeons in 1892, and received a doctorate from Trinity in 1894. During his undergraduate days he became intensely interested in the development of uses of electricity, and even during these years he contributed significantly to the field of electro-therapeutics. The therapeutic value of ionization, the breaking up of a substance into its constituent ions, was under discussion and he did considerable experimental work of value; he also worked on other electrical aids for dentistry. Then in 1895 Röntgen, a German physicist, made the discovery of x-rays for which his name became famous. Within a year Frank Price had constructed the first x-ray machine manufactured in Canada, though it is said that one was earlier imported to Montreal. Together with one of his brothers, who was in the manufacturing business, he devised a process of adding lead salts to rubber to make protective aprons and gloves for x-ray operators. He had already been appointed, upon graduation, to the staff of the Toronto school, as instructor and later as professor of electro-therapeutics, and in 1900 the school decided to buy its own x-ray machine. Without patterns to guide him, Price manufactured virtually all the electrical appliances in use in dental offices today, though they were in some cases markedly different in form from their modern counterparts. Among these appliances were controlled heaters for air, water, and wax, and cautery, sterilizer, and other devices, all of practical use. All of these he donated freely to the school, without thought of recompense. He was a popular speaker at dental meetings, greatly in advance of his times, for electricity had not yet been installed in dental offices. A note in the record of a meeting held in 1893 is significant: 'Evidently, the members did not think electricity had much connection with the practice of dentistry. The members did not seem to be very well-up on the subject and there was little discussion.'

By any standard of measurement, Frank Price was a great contributor to dental progress. His activities were not confined to electricity and he took an increasing interest in developing knowledge of the relationship between nutrition and dental caries. (A younger brother, Weston A. Price, DDS, MB SC, of Cleveland, a well known pioneer in this field, became president of the American Dental Association.) As the son of a Methodist lay preacher, Frank Price was a real humanitarian. All during the depression years he ground, packaged, and delivered a weekly source of fresh vitamin B to over one hundred poor families in co-operation with his friend, Sir Joseph Flavelle. At the time of his death in 1937, the Toronto newspapers paid glowing tribute to him, stating that his heart was set on the betterment of humanity, not on making money or an exclusive name for himself.[13]

According to papers presented at dental meetings, Peter Brown of

Montreal, of whom more will be said later, was a leader in the introduction of electricity into the dental office. Brown laid no claim to inventive genius, but recognized early the advantages and was instrumental in convincing dentists of the benefits of electricity. At every opportunity, either at dental meetings or as a teacher on the staff of the newly-formed Montreal dental school, he strongly advocated the use of electrical devices in the dental office as they became available.

Of other improvements, none had greater influence than the publication of the research findings of G.V. Black of Chicago on cavity preparation (1891) and balanced alloys (1895). He placed cavity preparation on a scientific basis, with emphasis on extension for prevention. Up to this time, alloys used for filling purposes were often of doubtful value: they tended to expand upon setting, which cracked the tooth, or to contract, which resulted in a leaking filling. By several years of experimentation, Black produced a balanced alloy which would neither expand nor contract, and which with little variation has stood the test of time. The beginnings of the use of baked porcelain for tooth restoration also occurred during this epoch, and the cast gold filling was in the experimental stage. The solder gold inlay was prepared by burnishing thin sheet

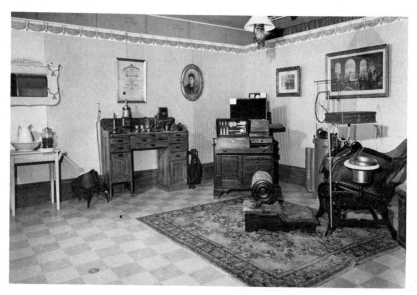

A dental operating room of the 1890s

gold into the cavity and then filling the shaped mold with solder. In general, local anaesthetics were in experimental use, but the solutions of cocaine being used often gave untoward results: at a meeting in 1895, J.B. Willmott denounced 'the sinful and unjustifiable practice of injecting anaesthetics' and he was probably right in relationship to what was being done at that time. Considerable technological advance occurred during the 1890s. Many refinements have occurred since, but most of the technical adjuncts used in the modern dental office either came into use or were in the experimental stage by the end of the nineteenth century.

Advancement in practice in this period depended almost entirely upon technological improvements and it is little wonder that dentists largely confined their attention to the development of their mechanical adjuncts. If a service was to be rendered, an efficient instrument was necessary. It was not until after the turn of the century that dentists were rather rudely awakened to certain facts concerning a health profession – that practice did not consist only of cements (sometimes called bone amalgams in early days), instruments, and techniques: a broadening concept in education and practice was essential, and the chief difference between a trade and a profession was that a profession gave more in service than was represented by the recompense received. These concepts were but faintly heard in the 1890s, but there were stirrings.

In 1892, the Montreal General Hospital appointed R. Hugh Berwick as staff dentist – the first Canadian dentist to receive a hospital appointment. Berwick had indentured with S.J. Andres of Montreal and obtained his Licentiate in Dental Surgery, following which he began the study of medicine at McGill University, graduating in 1891. He then decided to confine his practice to oral surgery, and in so doing may have been, by modern interpretation, the first specialist among dentists in Canada.[14] Berwick was recognized as one of the early brilliant men in dentistry. Unfortunately he died at twenty-six years of age from tuberculosis, said to have been the result of over-exertion in study. This appointment marks the beginning of a lasting relationship of dentistry with the Montreal General Hospital. J.S. Ibbottson was appointed to succeed him.

During this period the Toronto School outgrew available rented quarters. The number of students increased from sixty-six in 1892 to one hundred and thirty-five in 1896 and passed the two hundred mark in 1897. In the meantime, the course had been increased from two to three years. The situation called for drastic action, and in meeting the emergency Ontario dentists exhibited one of their finest hours. With strong support from the profession, the Ontario Board purchased a lot on College street, the eastern part of the land where the Toronto General Hospital now stands. Plans were devised for a sizeable building (two storeys 106 × 50 feet with basement) which was completed and opened with elaborate ceremonies on 1 October 1896. It was a financial venture of some magnitude for the time, amounting to approximately $50,000. No assistance from government or other source was received or contemplated: the profession accepted the full responsibility. The architect's description of the building emphasized modernity. While the profession is said to have worked as one man in accomplishing the project, the record shows that Dean J.B. Willmott and Henry T. Wood were the responsible leaders.

The Father of Public Health Dentistry in Canada was John C.G. Adams of Toronto, a man with a missionary zeal for dentistry. After completing his indentureship with an older brother, W. Case Adams, he opened practice in 1874. He was a man of strong convictions, great tenacity of purpose, unusual foresight, and simple Christian faith. Soon he became convinced that the then-current emphasis of dentistry was wrongly placed on dentures. The proper emphasis he felt, was to *preclude*

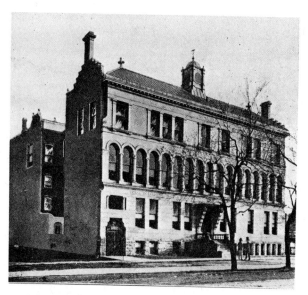

The Royal College of Dental Surgeons at 93 College Street, Toronto, built by Ontario dentists and opened in 1896

the need for artificial dentures by preventing diseases of the teeth among children. With the courage of his convictions, after qualifying, he founded a free dental hospital for poor children, naming it Christ's Dental Educational Institute.[15] The name indicates his missionary spirit and portends the emphasis on health education which was to come in later years, but in his day he struggled alone. He was not the type of man who pursued his conviction fractionally. Adams operated the free hospital for twenty-five years, during which he invested in it everything and it was said that no poor child in Toronto went without dental care. The picture of the hospital shows a sizeable three storey building which he had purchased with no money other than his own. Its end was tragic. Adams had a verbal understanding with the city authorities that the hospital was to be considered a charitable institution, but suddenly in 1899 the city seized the building and its contents for back taxes. Adams could not raise the demanded money. The newspapers took up his cause and the Toronto Dental Society made protest to the City Council, all to no avail.

In the meantime, Adams had written a 152-page book, *School Children's Teeth: Their Universally Unhealthy and Neglected Condition*, probably the first to be written on this subject. He also published a

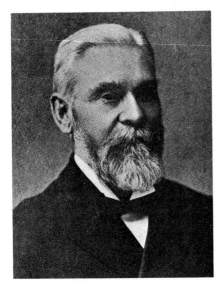

John Gennings Curtis Adams
(1839–1922)

pamphlet of sixteen pages for public distribution. Ironically, 5,000 copies of his book were seized by the city in closing his hospital. Fortunately, the influence of this one man, who had sacrificed so much, was destined to increase rapidly in adversity.

In 1896, Adams wrote, with documentary evidence respecting the condition of children's teeth, to the Ontario Board of Health. The communication was accompanied by a strong resolution from the Toronto Dental Society. The Toronto Trades and Labour Council also submitted a resolution to the government, requesting that action be taken to provide systematic dental health inspection of children in the public schools. The Board of Health set up a committee to consider the communication from Adams, and this committee produced a lengthy report. In essence, it recommended that municipalities appoint dental inspectors who would periodically visit the schools, examine pupil's teeth, and advise the children's parents what course to pursue. It was only a short time thereafter before the City of Toronto was spending $30,000 a year to replace Adam's hospital, which the city had closed because of $200 in back taxes. Adams had not only won public support but also had altered the concept of professional service. As time progressed, his views on preventive dentistry were accepted and adopted throughout Canada.

The Adams family has long played a notable part in the development of Canadian dentistry. An elder brother, W. Case Adams, began practising dentistry in Toronto during the early 1850s and is said to have trained more dentists by apprenticeship, including his brother and J.B. Willmott, than any other man. J. Franklin Adams, a son of J.G. Adams, conducted a most creditable practice in Toronto for forty-eight years and made many worthy contributions, among them the discovery of the famous 'Adams N & I Treatment' for purulent gum diseases that became widely used in Canada and abroad. His son, G.A. Cameron Adams, graduated in 1933, established practice in Toronto, and has served on the staff of the dental school. In 1965, J.R. Adams, son of G.A.C. Adams, extended the family profession to a fourth generation for the first time in Canada. A year later, 1966, the Bruce family of Kincardine, Ontario, became the second fourth-generation family of Canadian dentists.

During the 1890s an economic depression occurred in Canada, caused chiefly by the high-protective McKinley Tariff which came into effect in the United States. Money became scarce and a cry of overcrowding was heard from all professions in Canada, particularly from medicine and dentistry. At the same time, as stated above, the number of students in dentistry was increasing rapidly. Numerous editorials on the subject of an over-stocked profession appeared in the *Journal* and the situation dominated discussion at meetings. As editor, Beers attacked the problem in his usual forthright manner. A sampling of his statements in editorials represents the thinking of the time. He wrote initially, 'It is evident that the business of making dentists is progressing too fast, and that the supply is already far beyond the demand.' In reference to the expansion of the Toronto school, he stated that 'there were 160 students and with Ontario fully supplied with dentists, nobody knew where they were going to practise when they graduated.' For Quebec, he said, 'there were more students indentured than there were licentiates practising.' He pointed to a result: 'We can keep quacks from geting a licence, but it is doubtful if we can keep licentiates from becoming quacks, or using quack methods.' If all this criticism affected the leaders who were establishing the new enlarged school building at Toronto, no such indication appears in the records. The need for increased dental services existed. The difficulty was economic. The other contributing factor was lack of public appreciation for dental services.

Doubtless, when the Dental Boards in Ontario and Quebec were formed, the elected dentists thought that with law to enforce their efforts, qualified dentists would be quickly recognized and the quacks would disappear. Twenty years later they were still facing the problem, even after strenuous and continuing efforts, but to a much lesser degree. Dentists in the other provinces found themselves in a similar position after gaining legislation, and a large percentage of time and effort was devoted to the problem in each case. However, the beginnings of scientific meetings also occurred in all provinces, and at these meetings presentations of high calibre for that time were made. The British Columbia Dental Association was formed in 1891, with T.J. Jones elected president and A.C. West as secretary. In his address, the President referred to a former informal organization, the British Columbia Dental Society, and stated that the time had come for formal organization. The program of the second annual meeting gives an impression of advanced ratiocination for the period. The following papers were read and discussed:[16]

President's Address　　T.J. Jones, LDS
Administration of Ether　　Lewis Hall, DDS
The Relation of Physician and Dentist　　J. Holmes, DDS
Extraction of Children's Teeth　　W.J. Quinlan, DDS

Orthodontia   A.E. Verrinder, MD, DDS
Oral Surgery   H.F. Verrinder, MD, DDS
Treatment of Teeth During Pregnancy   A.R. Baker, DDS
Use of Electric Mallet (clinic)   A.R. Baker, DDS

In the Atlantic provinces, scientific meetings were arranged by the newly formed organizations on an annual basis. In 1898, the first joint meeting of these provinces was held at Digby. All of this was a giant stride forward from the individualistic secrecy which had dominated the attitude of the great majority of dentists. La Société d'Ontologie de Montréal and the Montreal Dental Club were formed, and the Toronto Dental Society became an active organization. Ottawa and several other centres formed local societies.

A scientific meeting was organized by the Ontario Dental Society in 1898 in celebration of the thirtieth anniversary of enactment of the Dental Act. Papers were presented summarizing the past, marking the iniquities of the present, and pointing out the objectives of the future. In his address, R.J. Husband of Hamilton gave portent of future activities in two statements: 'I believe we should extend our limits and I look hopefully to the time when we shall have a Dominion Association Meeting in different parts of the Dominion'; and, 'Individual members of the profession are responsible for the wide-spread ignorance and misinformation about the dental affairs which prevail everywhere.'

One of the most moving speeches during this decade was delivered by H.C. Wetmore in his presidential address before the New Brunswick Dental Society in 1897. 'It would be presumption on my part to recite the events, which to dentists, will appear as most important, when the doings of this period come to be crystallized into the history of the future. With them, we are all familiar. And with that noble band of apostles, the best years of whose lives were spent, and are being spent, in their endeavours to fathom the mysteries of our restricted specialty, or with those geniuses of mechanism and art, who have taught us to supply the deficiencies nature has oftentimes been guilty of in her handiwork, or to reproduce parts which man in his negligence or inability to preserve, have become useless or defunct – we, too, are familiar. Those sturdy veterans are aged and are aging. Many, too many, of those old familiar faces have already completed their last experiment, written their last treatise, and have departed to that bourn from which no traveller returneth.'[17]

The end of a century is a time of assessment and prognostication.

Canada consisted of seven provinces and an immense territory between Manitoba and British Columbia, with a total population of slightly over five million. Seventy-one per cent of the people lived in Ontario and Quebec, twelve per cent west of Ontario, and less than a million in the Atlantic Provinces. Of the cities, the two largest were Montreal with 267,730 people, and Toronto with 208,400. There were about 1,300 qualified dentists for the whole country, of whom 186 were in Quebec and 984 in Ontario.[18]

A most heartening aspect of the time was the fact that new and strong voices were arising within the profession and leadership appeared assured. Frank Woodbury, of Halifax, was beginning to be heard across the country and eventually became known as the Dean of Canadian Dentists. Each province had active men of leadership calibre who were devoting zeal and energy toward the advancement of the profession. Of the old guard, George Beers was to die within a year and J.B. Willmott was to give another fifteen years of service.

8

National organization
1900-1904

Two of the principal external features which contribute to the advancement of a profession are increased population and buoyant economic conditions. During the early years of the new century, some two million immigrants from Britain, Germany, Scandinavia, the Balkans, Russia, and the United States came to Canada as a result of federal government advertising, free homesteads, and assisted passages. This meant the coming of age of the Prairie provinces. From the southern part of the North-West Territories the provinces of Saskatchewan and Alberta were created in 1905. Much to the chagrin of Calgary, Edmonton became the capital of the latter, and after two years of wrangling, Regina won the parliament buildings of Saskatchewan. This action completed the political organization of Canada into provinces until 1949, when Newfoundland became the tenth province. Across the country, the population increased by fifty per cent to over seven million, in a short period.

Bread was five cents a loaf and milk five cents a quart. Coal sold for $4.50 a ton and $15 a month was good rent for a house. You could buy a ticket for twenty-one restaurant meals for $2.75, although in at least one restaurant there was a sign warning customers that a napkin would not be provided to anyone ordering a meal for under 15 cents. Women's chemises were featured in newspaper advertisements for 25 cents, and dress goods for 15 cents a yard. Meat was 6 to 12 cents a pound, according to cut. Skilled labourers in the construction trade received wages of $12 and common labourers from $8 to $10 a week. All of this was reflected in dental practice, with extractions at 25 to 50 cents, gold foil fillings at $2, and complete dentures at $10.

Canadian dentistry suffered one of its most grievous losses on 26 December 1900, when W. George Beers of Montreal died at fifty-nine years of age. For the advancement of his profession, his efforts knew no bounds. Outside the profession, he was widely known as a patriot, a sportsman, and a supporter of every good cause. The newspapers of the time, not only of his own city but across the country, devoted much space to extolling his virtues on a wide horizon. A booklet about him written by W.K. McNaught of Toronto, an industrialist and a member of the Ontario Legislature, appeared shortly after his death and was widely distributed across Canada. Seldom has any man received greater unmitigated praise and, as noted earlier, his name continues to appear in print to the present day. His appearance and personality were concisely described by McNaught:[1]

Dr Beers was no ordinary man. Of medium size, but admirably proportioned and with a face singularly resembling that of the lamented General Gordon of Sudan fame, he had a personality that was at once striking and attractive. One could not be in his company long before becoming impressed with the fact that he was not only a gentleman in the truest sense of the word, but a man of scholarly attainments, who had seen much of the world and whose opinions on most subjects were the results of personal convictions, rather than derived from others.

A large square granite stone marks the grave of this outstanding Canadian dentist in the Mount Royal Cemetery in Montreal. His influence still is felt. Among his contributions was that of his dental library to the Royal College of Dental Surgeons of Ontario – undoubtedly the largest dental library in Canada at the time, consisting of some four hundred volumes. The library was housed in the Toronto school and formed the nucleus of the large library collection now possessed by the Faculty of Dentistry, University of Toronto.

The death of Beers left the editorship of the *Dominion Dental Journal* vacant. Fortunately for the future of the *Journal*, a young man, Albert E. Webster of Toronto, was appointed editor, a position he was to hold for thirty-five years. Beers' position as dean of the Montreal school proved considerably more difficult to fill. Following his resignation in 1897, Stephen Globensky was appointed but occupied the position for only a little over a year. He was followed by his brother, J.G. Globensky, for one session. W.J. Kerr was dean for the session 1900–01, and William J. Giles was dean during the next session. Peter Brown, a prominent Montreal dentist, was appointed in 1902 and remained dean until 1905, when the school was closed.

It is evident that a good deal of dissatisfaction arose at the school respecting the relationship with the University of Bishop's College. The effort to teach in both French and English also had not proven very successful. The Quebec Board consequently held new discussions with both McGill and Laval Universities, which culminated in 1904 with agreements whereby both universities agreed to undertake formal dental education, in the case of Laval at its Montreal branch (which became l'Université de Montréal in 1920). The progress of this change was hastened by the fact that Bishop's Medical College in Montreal ceased to exist and was joined with the Medical Faculty of McGill University in 1905.[2]

Both new schools opened in the fall of 1905, and the Quebec Board abolished the Dental College of the Province of Quebec. Arrangements were necessary, however, for the teaching of practical dentistry. For this purpose the Quebec Board rented clinic quarters over Sax's clothing store at the corner of St Lawrence and St Catherine Streets. Later, in 1906, the clinic was moved to space in the newly erected *La Patrie* newspaper building. In reality, that is to say, the Quebec Board continued to provide for the teaching of practical dentistry until the universities were able to make proper arrangements for doing so. In 1906, the clinic for McGill students was moved to the Montreal General Hospital, where clinical instruction has been given to the present. Laval students remained until 1909, when the equipment was sold to l'Université Laval for $450, as recorded in the Dental Board minutes. The details of the transfer of the teaching of practical dentistry from the Quebec Board to the universities are difficult to delineate. The participation of the Dental Board, beyond providing space and equipment for the clinic, is not clear. In any event, McGill had taken over complete control of dental students by 1906 and Laval had done so by 1909.

The McGill dental clinic made use of the large morgue facilities of the Montreal General Hospital. Up to this time, extensive morgues had been necessary to meet the tragic results of large-scale epidemics of smallpox. The fight for the introduction of vaccination, which took place in practically all communities, was particularly intense and severe in Montreal; and the death of a prominent young Montreal dentist, John H. Samuel, while not resulting in the adoption of compulsory vaccination, did create a turning point in the battle for this public health measure. Gradually, vaccination won out and smallpox subsided; extensive morgue facilities were no longer necessary and could be converted to other uses.

At both universities, the dental course was established as four years in duration, the length adopted by the Royal College of Dental Surgeons in 1903. The incorporation of the dental schools within the university structure differed considerably. At Laval, the dental school became a division of the university with Eudore Dubeau as dean, a position he held for some forty years. At McGill, the dental school became a department of the Faculty of Medicine. The initial McGill announcement stated: 'This department is not independent, but it is a section of the Medical Faculty.'[3] The same announcement listed instructors in the dental department but did not indicate a head of the department. The name of Peter Brown appeared first on the list. Previously he had been dean of the Bishop's school, and he has been referred to as head of the department at McGill, but this is not specifically stated. Dentistry did not become a full faculty at McGill until 1920.

From the beginning, Laval conferred the degree of Doctor of Dental Surgery, but McGill refused to do so. The first calendar issued by McGill stated that upon completion of the course the degree of Master of Dental Surgery (MDS) would be conferred. It was found that a master's degree could not be conferred, however, and the calendar for the following year offered the degree of Graduate in Dental Surgery (GDS). In 1908, McGill finally announced the degree of Doctor of Dental Surgery (DDS). Doubtless this decision was influenced by a loophole quickly discovered by the students. The University of Bishop's College, even though it had stopped giving courses in Montreal, had not relinquished the right to confer degrees in medicine and dentistry, and McGill dental students found that by registering at Bishop's they could qualify for the doctorate, which they proceeded to do. Only six GDS degrees were ever conferred by McGill, all in 1906, and three of these were later converted to doctorates. One went to George Lynch Cameron, who became a prominent Canadian dentist.

In this context, the cases of George L. Cameron and George S. Cameron are interesting. Both men began their studies at Bishop's, and had completed two years of the course when the school was closed and they were transferred to McGill. There they were informed that they had to begin again in the first year. George L. dutifully did so and after graduation practised at Swift Current, Saskatchewan, for many years, becoming a distinguished member of the profession. George S. refused

McGill's condition as insulting, and went to the United States to complete his education. On his return to Montreal, he was granted permission to write his licensure examination and performed so impressively that he was invited to teach at McGill; for many years he was one of the most prominent dentists in the city.

This period also saw the creation of a national dental association. As early as 1889 Beers had published an editorial advocating the formation of a Dominion Dental Society. In his usual forthright manner, he had pointed out the weaknesses of individual provincial policies and the advantages of concerted action on a national basis. He continued his advocacy for a national dental organization but unfortunately did not live long enough to see its consummation.

Frank Woodbury of Halifax, who was secretary of the Nova Scotia dental body, initiated a movement in 1893 for reciprocity between the provincial dental boards. In some detail, he pointed out the similarities and differences in licencing requirements of the various boards. The differences which did exist were minor ones, and with slight alterations reciprocity could be achieved. The Nova Scotia Dental Association unanimously supported the proposal and resolved to work toward its attainment. Discussions by correspondence and personal conversation between provincial representatives continued, and grew. Both Beers and Webster gave strong editorial support, and many of the dental organizations adopted favourable resolutions.

For a period of ten years, enthusiasm for the organization of the profession on a national basis increased in every province. S.W. McInnis of Brandon, F.A. Godsoe of Saint John, Frank Woodbury of Halifax, J.S. Bagnall of Charlottetown, W.D. Cowan of Regina, R. Nash of Victoria, F.A. Stevenson of Montreal, and J.B. Willmott of Toronto were among the strongest advocates. Credit for taking the vital final step rightfully belongs to the Quebec Dental Association, whose secretary, Eudore Dubeau, mailed a letter to every dentist in Canada containing these significant sentences:[4]

Every dentist who can rise above mere local or provincial affairs in our country, and has thought about the immense advantages to be gained by the nationalization of the dental profession, should unhesitatingly give the idea his support. The legal representatives of the profession in the various provinces have agreed to work toward giving dentistry a national character.

The way seems to be prepared for the first step towards the goal. The

Quebec Dental Association, together with one representative from each of the provinces, have undertaken to organize a meeting in Montreal, September 16th, 1902 ...

F.A. Stevenson was president of the Quebec Association at the time and an outstanding dentist. He had graduated from the Harvard University Dental School in 1888 and practised in Montreal until his death in 1934. During his lifetime, Stevenson held practically every possible position in his profession, was honoured by his fellow practitioners in many ways, and served on the teaching staff of the McGill school. With the unanimous support of the Quebec Association, he and Dubeau organized the meeting. Stevenson presided at the meeting and hence became the first president.

The attendance at this meeting in 1902 was remarkable. Some 344 dentists were present, nineteen per cent of the dentists in Canada at the time. All provinces and the North-West Territories were represented. The meeting ran for three days and enthusiasm was great. Both the lengthy scientific program and the business sessions indicated great care in preparation. From the business sessions resulted two new national dental organizations – the Canadian Dental Association and the Dominion Dental Council, both created with great unanimity.

It is evident that a great deal of work had preceded the meeting, for each delegate was presented when he registered with a copy of the proposed constitution and by-laws of a Canadian Dental Association. Also a code of ethics was presented, which was a slightly amended version of that adopted by the National Dental Association (later renamed American Dental Association). Prepared papers on various phases of national organization were presented from each province, each expressing approval of the objective. After discussion and minor amendments, the constitution and by-laws, together with the code of ethics, were adopted.

The first action taken by the newly formed Association was the adoption of a strongly worded resolution requesting the several corporate bodies to appoint one member each to a Dominion Dental Council. These appointees were to formulate a scheme for establishing a nation-wide qualification for the practice of dentistry which would be acceptable to the several licensing boards. Their recommendations were to be reported to the next meeting of the Association. For the first time, there was something less than full unanimity, however. The Quebec representatives stated that while they were not personally opposed, the proposal for reciprocity of licence was reaching for an ideal too quickly. On the other hand, the president of the British Columbia Board of Examiners, T.J. Jones, who was unable to attend, sent a letter to the meeting in praise of Dominion registration. All the other provinces welcomed the objective enthusiastically.

This meeting was the first time Canadian dentists had come together, and many other subjects of mutual interest were discussed. Dental health education for the public was one predominant theme. Both Ontario and Nova Scotia had made some progress toward public education, and following the meeting efforts were initiated in other provinces patterned on their experience. The need for a dental corps was the other principal subject of discussion. The South African War (1899–1902) had concluded only a few weeks before the meeting. In all, about 7,300 Canadians had crossed the ocean to fight in it, and soon after their arrival overseas letters had been received in Canada telling of their sufferings from defective teeth. As a result, two dentists, David Henry Baird of Ottawa and Eugene Lemieux of Montreal, were taken on the army's strength in 1900 and sent to South Africa, where they served until May 1902.[5] No record exists respecting their equipment but it is known that they rendered extractions and emergency services and presumably they took their own equipment with them. Baird and Lemieux were the first Canadians to serve as dental surgeons in a military field of action. The first recorded proposal for military dentistry was made by the Eastern Ontario Dental Association in 1900 in a strong resolution that provision be made in the militia for the appointment of dental surgeons to the forces. Other dental organizations quickly forwarded similar resolutions to the authorities. The government's replies were favourable but said that no provision existed for the appointment of such officers. Ira Bower, an Ottawa dentist, had been most active in this effort and he presented a paper at the first national meeting summarizing the position. A supporting resolution was adopted, setting up a national committee with Bower as chairman, which became one of the most active committees of the newly-formed Association. In view of later developments, the wording of the resolution, 'favour the adoption by the Militia Department of provision for a regular army dental staff which shall be a *distinct* branch of the service,' is interesting.

The enthusiasm engendered at the founding meeting was great and delegates returned home feeling that real progress had been made. Previous to the formation of the Canadian Dental Association, the *Dominion Dental Journal* had been the profession's only unifying force. In a large country like Canada, geography and finance are the principal enemies to be overcome in national organizations. A third factor faced by the CDA was the strength of its membership – approximately 1,310 dentists stretched across a thin ribbon of over 4,000 miles. These conditions were considered realistically and it was decided that only biennial meetings were possible.

The second meeting of the Canadian Dental Association took place at Toronto in September 1904. In his presidential address, J.B. Willmott summarized the position of dentistry in Canada.[6]

The organization of the Canadian Dental Association marked, to some extent, the time of completion of the preliminary stage in the development of the dental profession in Canada. Provincial and local societies had been formed in every province. For the protection of the public against the injury to the public health which would result from unskilful dental operations, each provincial legislature had passed laws requiring a good degree of professional education and skill. The corporate bodies constituted under these laws had organized the profession and fixed a high standard for admission in the several provinces. Dental schools had been established in Quebec and Ontario, with capacity for the education of the dental students of the Dominion. From small beginnings, the Dominion Dental Journal had grown to be a large and influential factor in maintaining and extending the credit of Canadian dentistry. What still was lacking was the bringing together of the results of the good work accomplished in the several provinces and making it effective in the development of dentistry throughout the Dominion.

The report of the committee on military dentistry was significant. The appointment of dental surgeons had been authorized on 2 July 1904, although the committee had been unsuccessful in securing an independent corps. The chairman, Ira Bower, had been persistent in gaining support for the objective and was to continue his effort for satisfactory arrangements: initial credit for the establishment of dental service in the Canadian forces rightfully belongs to him.

The process of organizing the Dominion Dental Council proved to be slower than anticipated. Meetings of the representatives of the provincial boards were held in both 1904 and 1905, with all provinces represented except British Columbia. The Quebec representatives stated that they could not report a firm decision from their Board, but other representatives reported affirmation. This meant that seven of the nine provinces were prepared to accept reciprocal agreements, although two provinces, Saskatchewan and Alberta, were in the process of formation and final affirmation would be necessary by each. The organizing committee, under the chairmanship of Frank Woodbury of Halifax, had performed a great deal of preparatory work. At the 1905 meeting held in Toronto, a very complete document containing the objects, rules, and standards, as well as the detailed operation, of the Council was presented. After discussion in detail, and with some amendments, this document was adopted as the constitution and by-laws. Harry R. Abbott of London was elected the first president, and W.D. Cowan of Regina became secretary. The first examinations were conducted in 1906; C.H. Juvet of Ottawa is the first in the register of recipients of the Dominion Dental Council Certificate.[7] The Council continued to serve the participating provinces for forty-five years, when it was succeeded by the National Dental Examining Board. Quebec did not join the agreement at any time, but for several years sent representatives to the meetings. On two occasions, British Columbia participated for a brief period. Under the reciprocal agreement, the holder of a Council Certificate was entitled to register for licence to practise in any participating province. The arrangement was a most sensible one which served initially to bring uniformity of qualification throughout Canada, and which continued to work to the advantage of both dentists and provincial licencing boards.

Owing to the small number of dentists in the west, it was difficult to hold satisfactory scientific meetings on a provincial basis during this period. At the annual meeting of the Manitoba Dental Association in January 1900, a decision was made to organize the Western Canada Dental Society. The first meeting of the new society was held in Winnipeg the following July. R.R. Dalgleish of Winnipeg was elected president and G.C. Mathison became secretary. This meeting proved successful, and while, as with most societies, some difficulties arose from time to time, the dentists in the provinces of Manitoba, Saskatchewan, and Alberta have continued to support their regional body at biennial meetings.

The idea still prevailed that all pertaining to the practice of dentistry must be kept within the confines of the dental office and performed by the dentist himself or in a minor way by a properly indentured student, but cracks were appearing in the wall. Already, as related earlier, the philosophy of secrecy had been attacked by dentists who wanted to employ assistants in their offices, and in spite of objections from the dental boards, such assistants were gradually making their appearance. At about the turn of the century, dental supply houses in both Toronto and Montreal conceived the idea of setting up laboratories to perform mechanical services for their clients. The dental boards reacted sharply; letters went to the supply houses stating that such laboratories must be closed, as they were engaged in the practice of dentistry without a licence. The laboratories ceased to operate. It should be explained that in those days the laboratory was an integral part of the dental office and of practice, and considered of vital importance. Although the board's attitude may seem reactionary today, to condone the establishment of dental laboratories outside of dental offices at the time was comparable to splitting dental practice in half. The employment of assistants and the laboratory affair were directly related. With few exceptions, the assistants employed were males and their main duties were in the laboratory. It was natural that gradually some of these men, trained by a dentist in his own office, would do the same work independently for several dentists. As a result, and in spite of the boards, by 1905 the commercial dental laboratory was well established in the cities. An editorial in the *Dominion Dental Journal* of that year confirmed that there was more money to be made in running a laboratory for the profession than in working on salary for a single dentist. Like so many alterations in the way of things, the change had an economic basis.

Study of the Canadian dental literature over many years reveals intensive discussions respecting the relationship of medicine and dentistry. The subject reached a crescendo around the turn of the century. Diverse views existed among the leaders of the profession. J.B. Willmott argued in his usual forthright manner that dentistry was *not* a specialty of medicine. Frank Woodbury stated that 'nothing should claim more attention than a study of our proper relation to the public at large, and the status of dental surgery among the specialties of medicine.'[8] The arguments dated back to the beginnings of dentistry, when in European countries it was considered a part of surgery. Men like John Hunter of England emphasized its biological aspects. When the first dental school was established at Baltimore, after an attempt to teach dentistry in the medical school there, it was settled that the practice of dentistry could not be taught in a medical school. Henceforth dentistry on the North American continent became independent, while in a dwindling number of European countries a medical course remains a prerequisite for its study. The adoption of an autonomous position brought rapid development to professional status. It also gave impetus to the invention of innumerable practical aids to practice in the form of instruments, materials, and techniques, accompanied by an ever-improving reputation. By the early 1900s, however, the pendulum had started to swing back toward the biological aspects of dentistry, and this caused men to think again in terms of the medical-dental relationship. The discussions continued; the situation was met over the years to the present by an increasing biological content in the dental curriculum.

Advertising was still the bane of the profession. There was an increasing interest in dentistry, indicated positively by the growing number of applicants to the schools. On the darker side were the commercial artifices employed by a certain class of men to whom moral suasion was a farce. Quacks and quack imitators made a point of challenging the world in general and reputable dentists in particular. Each one publicly declared that he was the only genuine and unadulterated genius in the profession; that he was the author of ideas which were old before he entered the profession; that he was the inventor of appliances which everybody else had the good sense not to use. These men utilized tricks of trade and theatrical superlatives with the objectives of circus advertisers.

Their methods took many forms. Their activities were, in the main, confined to the larger cities, although the large newspaper advertisements, handbills, and cards affected the whole profession. Among them were the Good Samaritan Dental Association, which placed large advertisements in Montreal newspapers in 1899 announcing in large type, that 'Tyranny is Dead' and 'Revolution has again Succeeded,' and promising among other items, perfect-fitting artificial teeth for $4.85 and gold fillings, 1000th fine, from $1.00. The Boston Dental Parlours also placed advertisements in the newspapers. In Toronto, the Toronto Painless Dental Parlours and department store dentistry became issues. In Montreal, a bookkeeper named Paquette established the 'Institute Dentaire Franco-American' and hired dentists, thus forming a company practice and advertising services at ridiculously low rates. Through court action, the Quebec Association finally succeeded in closing this organization. New amendments to the Dental Acts were sought and obtained to deal with the problem. However, as soon as one door was closed, another was opened by some ingenious device, and the battle continued for two more decades. In retrospect, it appears regrettable that the profession had to spend so much time, effort and money in overcoming a situation created primarily by a small minority.

The last great gold rush on the Pacific slope began with the discovery of gold on the Klondike, a tributary of the Yukon River. Rapidly, men

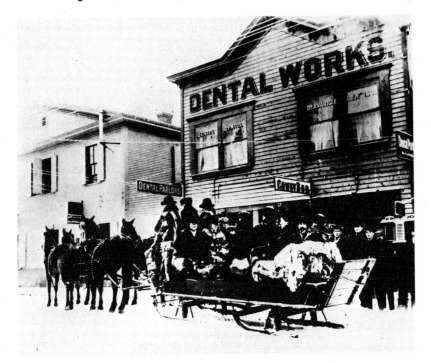

The first dental office at Dawson City, Yukon

came from all over the world to the area, overcoming tremendous difficulties in transportation. In 1897 the population of Dawson City was 1,500, a year later it had increased to 25,000. Among the newcomers were a few dentists, who arrived initially seeking wealth other than by practise. The first to actually establish a dental office was Antoine Avaricle, who exhibited a certificate stating that he was a member of La Societé Dentaire de Paris. Avaricle set up his office over the Comey Bar, which was probably a good location in the mining community as far as traffic was concerned. By 1900, the main rush was over and decline had set in, but other smaller deposits continued to be discovered. Avaricle moved his office to Granville, some seventy-five miles south of Dawson, and there Francis George Berton apprenticed with him. A short time later, Avaricle left for parts unknown. Berton carried on the practice for a period in order to supply the community with a dental service, then turned to other occupations. Twenty years later, the total population of the enormous Yukon Territory was 5,000 souls; by 1930 fewer than a thousand were living at

Dawson. During this interval over a dozen dentists are known to have practised in the area for varying lengths of time. Surprisingly, among them was one lady, Nanette Finlay Clay, who is listed in 1911. When the last qualified dentist, A.W. Faulkner, left Dawson in 1925, F.G. Berton bought his equipment and maintained the practice until other dentists appeared. His son, the author and broadcaster, Pierre Berton, states that: 'My mouth and that of my sister's, all those years, seemed to be constantly full of plaster of paris as my father practised taking impressions to fit people for dentures.' The elder Berton made no claim to be a qualified dentist. However, he filled a need and his services were greatly appreciated. Of the other dentists who practised in the Yukon during this era, all except two or three exhibited academic qualifications of some kind, but none were Canadian graduates.

Canadian dentistry was reaching a stage of maturity with many indications of increased recognition. The future appeared bright. In his presidential address at the annual meeting of the Ontario Dental Society in 1904, R.E. Sparks of Kingston expressed the attitude prevailing among dentists:[9]

As I look over the horizon, I see dawning great possibilities for those entering our profession at the present time. The x-rays, the microscope, the fluoroscope, the development of bacteriology, the introduction of electricity, the recognition of the reaction of general to local diseases, and the invention of new instruments and appliances, are doing wonders in the prevention, diagnosis and treatment of dental ills. But, I believe our knowledge of these subjects is but in its infancy. The young men who enter upon a scientific study of dentistry, and who carry their study and research into their practices after graduation, have opportunities of becoming famous, and of making ours one of the grandest, because one of the most beneficial of professions.

9
Oral sepsis
1905-1909

In the Atlantic provinces young men found it necessary to go to Boston or some other centre in the United States in order to study dentistry. This was expensive, and a deterrent to increasing the number of practitioners in the area. Early in the century, the Nova Scotia Dental Association, under the leadership of Frank Woodbury, initiated a movement for the establishment of a dental school. Consultations were held with the New Brunswick Dental Society and the Prince Edward Island Dental Association. Unanimous agreement was reached that a school should be founded, and that it should be located in Halifax with a relationship to Dalhousie University.

In response to that initiative, the Nova Scotia Legislature at its 1906–7 session passed an Act establishing the Maritime Dental College. Through hearty co-operation of Dalhousie University and the Halifax Medical College, an agreement was formulated. Under it, Dalhousie supplied the dental infirmary, laboratories, and lecture rooms, together with adequate staff for the teaching of chemistry, physics, and biology. The Halifax Medical College agreed to teach anatomy, physiology, histology, bacteriology, and materia medica to the dental students, and to supply necessary laboratory facilities for those subjects. Dalhousie established a Faculty of Dental Surgery to examine candidates for the degree of Doctor of Dental Surgery. Dental students were accorded necessary privileges in the Victoria General Hospital. A four-year course began 1 September 1908.

Leaders in the provinces of Quebec and Ontario, where the struggle for proper dental education had been so arduous and lengthy, must have read with amazement of such achievements in so short a time. Yet the accomplishment was not as easy as it may appear. As always in establishing a school, financial difficulties constituted a major stumbling-block. The teaching of dental subjects remained the obligation of the dentists themselves, and, since the school was designed to serve the Atlantic region as a whole, dentists from New Brunswick, Prince Edward Island, Nova Scotia, and Newfoundland served as members of the initial staff. The Nova Scotia Dental Association made a grant to the maximum of its ability, and in addition each member of the Dental Board contributed fifty dollars, a sizeable amount for that period. The ownership of the Maritime Dental College remained in the hands of the Nova Scotia Dental Association, and as much financial support as possible was freely granted in each succeeding year. This arrangement prevailed until 1912, when both the Maritime Dental College and the Halifax Medical College ceased to exist, under an agreement whereby Dalhousie University took over complete teaching in both faculties. Thus, Dalhousie was the first university in Canada to establish a fully integrated faculty of dentistry.

Frank Woodbury was appointed the first dean of the college, a position he held until his death in 1922. He had been the first registrar of the Dental

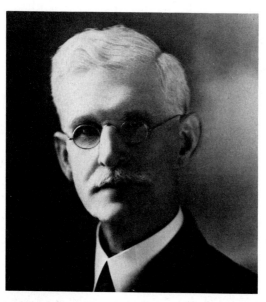

Frank Woodbury, DDS, LLD, Dean of the Faculty of
Dentistry, Dalhousie University, 1908–22

THE WOODBURY FAMILY IN DENTISTRY

FRANCIS WOODBURY (1813–1852)
a farmer in Annapolis County, NS

HIBBERT WOODBURY (1842–19'3)

apprenticed in Massachusetts
graduated Philadelphia Dental
College, 1877
practised at Halifax, 1878–1913
charter member, NS Dental Association
a founder, Maritime Dental College
professor of prosthetics (1904–12)

FRANK WOODBURY (1853–1922)

graduated Pennsylvania Dental
College, 1878
practised at Halifax, 1878–1922
first registrar, NS Dental Board
president, NS Dental
Association, 1898
a founder of Dominion
Dental Council
dean, Maritime Dental
College, 1908–12
dean, Faculty of Dentistry,
Dalhousie University, 1912–22
president, Canadian Dental
Association, 1918
Hon. LLD from Dalhousie
University, 1920
first president, Dental Faculties
Association, 1920

WILLIAM W. WOODBURY (1882–1967)

graduated, Philadelphia Dental
College, and
opened general practice,
Halifax, 1908
orthodontics at Halifax, 1920
professor of orthodontics, 1910–52
dean at Dalhousie University, 1935–47
president, Canadian Dental
Association, 1940–2
Hon. LLD from Dalhousie
University, 1953

RALPH H. WOODBURY (1884–1924)

graduated, Philadelphia
Dental College, 1908
on staff, Maritime Dental
College, 1909–24

KARL WOODBURY (1893–1946)

graduated, Dalhousie
University, 1915
served in Canadian Army
Dental Corps, 1916–19
lecturer at Dalhousie Dental
Faculty for several years

Board and later was elected president of the Nova Scotia Dental Association. The groundwork for the establishment of the Dominion Dental Council was done by him, and later he became president of the Canadian Dental Association. Comparable in his home province to Beers in Quebec and Willmott in Ontario, he also contributed so greatly on the national level that he became known as the Dean of Canadian Dentists. Indeed, the Woodbury family were all intimately connected with the development of the profession. Each also was extremely active in lay enterprises, particularly those of religious and related charitable organizations.

Over the years, New Brunswick had benefited from some of Canada's earliest resident dentists and had experienced one of the country's most difficult legislatures. A.J. McAvenney described both developments in a short historical summary.[1] In it he stated that Mr Rath, surgeon dentist, had established an office at Saint John in 1823. Itinerant dentists had visited that city earlier. Other residents, in the main of Loyalist stock from the United States, had followed Rath, spreading to Fredericton and other municipalities. The number of dentists increased slowly, but when they organized in 1890 as the New Brunswick Dental Society they proved to be a progressive group, which from the beginning carried on scientific programs at its annual meetings. Much of their leaders' time, however, was consumed in dealing with the legislature. Both the Quebec and Ontario associations had tribulations with their respective legislatures, which over-ruled the Boards and granted licences for practice to unqualified individuals, but this problem appears to have been more severe and lasted longer in New Brunswick than in any other province.

During the early period, a considerable number of strong leaders developed in New Brunswick on both provincial and national levels. Among them, Frank A. Godsoe, who served as registrar and secretary from 1891 to 1931, made an outstanding contribution. He lived a long life, dying at the age of one hundred in 1962. Godsoe had a rare professional breadth of vision for his day and left a lasting memory of altruism. The first registered dentist in New Brunswick was J.M. Magee, who graduated from Pennsylvania College of Dental Surgery in 1883 and immediately became active in the development of his profession. After serving in many capacities in his own province he broadened his activities, becoming a charter member and later president of both the Canadian Dental Association and the Dominion Dental Council. One of his colleagues, C.A. Murray, is credited with successfully carrying through the effort to secure a Dental Act in 1890 after several earlier attempts had failed. A.J. McAvenney, the first president of the New Brunswick Dental Society, and George O. Hannah, the first president of the Saint John Dental Society, both played important parts in establishing the profession in their province. All possessed high objectives together with the stamina to work consistently toward achievement.

New Brunswick also produced the greatest showman dentist ever known on this continent in the person of Edgar Randolph Parker, better known by his own description as Painless Parker. While for over half a century his name appeared from time to time in dental literature, for the most part it was in relation to legal actions brought about by the profession against him. He attracted great publicity, however, in the lay press.[2] Parker almost reached perfection as a showman, but dentists who knew him also admitted that he was a capable practitioner for his era, which stretched to modern times. A brief outline of his career suggests the story of others who operated in perhaps a less expansive style.

Painless Parker was born at Tynemouth Creek, a small village in New Brunswick; in his youth he tried to become a minister, but was expelled from both Acadia University and the Baptist Seminary at St. Martin's, NB. How he became interested in dentistry is not known, but he gained

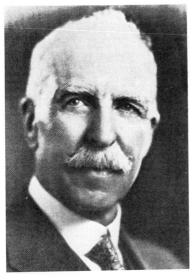

James M. Magee, DDS, first registered
dentist in New Brunswick

admission to the New York College of Dentistry for part of a course. Then he was expelled for practising outdoor dentistry while a student. He was next admitted to the Philadelphia Dental College, where he graduated in 1891. On his return to his native province, he obtained a licence and established practice in a small community, St Martin's, renting the second chair in a one-man barber shop. Although he exhibited great respectability by faithfully carrying a large Bible under his arm to church each Sunday, his practice did not thrive. He turned to other methods. From this point forward, Parker relied upon circus adjuncts to attract patients, and the stories of his activities are legion. By means of handbills and all other available forms of advertising, he drew the crowds to free street-corner shows with chorus girls, clowns, brass bands, and many other attractions. During his early years, his income was derived from so-called painless extractions. One of his early methods was to have a man with a bugle stand behind the patient and blow a blast at a given signal: this distracted the patient just when the tooth was coming out.

Except for one or two short intervals, Parker spent little time in New Brunswick. He set up shop in Brooklyn, NY, and engaged a tightwire artist to traverse a wire stretched across the street to his office window. As far as the crowds below were aware, the artist entered the window and had a tooth extracted painlessly every hour. Free of charge, and for advertising purposes only, he inserted diamonds in the anterior teeth of the great prize fighter, Bob Fitzsimmons. In a few years, he had thirty-six dentists on his payroll in the Brooklyn and Manhattan area. In his prosperity he took to wearing a swallowtail coat and cultivated a Vandyke beard. As most of the many articles published about him were based upon his own statements, often extremely boastful, it is difficult to separate truth from fiction. Financially, he was successful, and when he decided to retire in New York, officially it was because of ill health. Perhaps a better reason was that the eastern states had been busy amending their dental legislation respecting advertising, thus creating difficulties for him. In any case he moved to California, where his retirement lasted only a few months. Within a few years, Parker had several offices in Los Angeles and gradually extended his offices in the cities along the west coast to twenty-seven, including one in Vancouver. Any attempt to enumerate his activities would demand much space. At one stage he bought a circus, and as ringmaster advertised the dentistry to be obtained in his offices. He also rented store windows and practised in the windows to attract crowds. To defeat the law that a dentist must practise under his own name, he had his name changed by

A GRAND
Free Open Air Concert

at 3 p. m., and 7 p. m., every day.

—CONSISTING OF—

VOCAL AND INSTRUMENTAL MUSIC.

TEETH EXTRACTED

Free of Charge, Without Pain,

By a perculiar method of his own, with

WHIPS, SWORDS, SPOONS AND INSTRUMENTS
OF HIS OWN INVENTION.

Amusing!
Interesting!
Entertaining!
Astonishing!

Nothing to corrupt the morals of the most refined or fastidious person in the City.

COME ONE AND ALL TO THE TENT,
ERECTED ON THE
Cor. UNION ST. AND CHIPMAN HILL,
OPPOSITE ODD FELLOWS' HALL.

Telegraph Press.

Handbill distributed by Edgar Randolph Parker ('Painless Parker,' king of the advertising dentists) in Saint John, NB, in 1896 court order to Painless Parker. He became an expert in defeating court actions against him, although he did not win them all.

Parker died in 1952 at eighty years of age. At one time, he boasted that he had practised in every province in Canada, but it has not been possible to obtain proof of this statement. He was a Canadian export contributed, without regret, by the dental profession to the United States. First and foremost he was a showman, who claimed to have done more to publicize dentistry than any other man. Perhaps this is true, but the difficulty lay in his methods. He claimed also to have brought dentistry to the poor, but examination of related finances shed doubt on this statement as well. The dental profession in North America has had a considerable number of advertisers; Parker was king of them all.

Some of the other individuals who attempted dentistry by means of circus-like performances carried on for a period, while others failed after brief efforts, probably due to lack of showmanship. None was able to succeed for long in Canada. Two examples of widely different types are 'Professor' Ashley and Madame Enault. The Original Professor Napoleon Ashley, The King of Dentists (according to his advertisements), roamed the Atlantic Provinces with his group of entertainers for a few years. He claimed to be from Montreal, but no record of him has been found at that city and the name used was likely a pseudonym. During one of his performances at Charlottetown in May 1880, he extracted teeth for a Mrs McDonald and later that night she bled to death. An immediate search for Ashley found that he had absconded. He was not heard of afterwards.[3]

A more peculiar case was that of Madame Enault, the only known woman in this category. In June 1882, 'Dr' and Madame Dufot Enault arrived in Montreal from Belgium on the transatlantic liner Helvetia. They posed in considerable style and a few days later Madame Enault left the Richelieu Hotel in a beautiful carriage pulled by three superb horses and escorted by twelve Mexican musicians. She paraded through town, putting on a show in Jacques Cartier Square before a large crowd of people. In her sales pitch she claimed to extract teeth without pain. She also had a panacea, referred to in newspaper accounts as 'Chinese Perfume,' which would cure practically any physical disability. In the course of a few weeks she extracted hundreds of teeth and distributed great quantities of her panacea. The physicians and dentists of Montreal reacted strongly, to such an extent that the Enaults left for Quebec City, where they repeated their performance with the same success. However, their stay in Quebec was shorter because, as the reports state, the dentists and physicians were able to gain the assistance of the clergy and the Enaults left suddenly. No further trace of them has been found.[4]

In the west, meanwhile, the political formation of Alberta and Saskatchewan necessitated the enactment of dental legislation in each new province. The first meeting of the dentists of Alberta was held 3–5 October 1905 with sixteen in attendance. The initial purpose was the formation of an organization. R.B. Sullivan (president), A.E. Aunger (secretary), C.F. Strong, R.C. McClure, and E.M. Doyle were elected members of the first Alberta Board. After reviewing available dental legislation and drafting a tentative bill, they applied to the legislature for enactment, and the Dental Law of Alberta was assented to 9 May 1906. The early minutes of the College of Dental Surgeons of Saskatchewan are lost. From other sources it is known that the first meeting of Saskatchewan dentists was held at approximately the same time as that in Alberta and that W.D. Cowan was elected president. Cowan and Lorenzo D. Keown were active members of the council of the college from the beginning and remained so for many years.

In form, the Act adopted in Saskatchewan in 1906 followed closely that which had existed in the North-West Territories, with appropriate alterations: it created the College of Dental Surgeons of Saskatchewan, retaining the same members of Council until their successors were elected. The Alberta Act created the Alberta Dental Association with provision for the election of a board of directors from its members. Both Acts stated that every person duly qualified and registered by the College of Dental Surgeons of the North-West Territories was automatically eligible for membership. With minor variations, the legislation was similar to that existing in the other provinces. In British Columbia, Saskatchewan, Ontario, and Quebec, the Acts established a college of dental surgeons; in Alberta, Manitoba, New Brunswick, Nova Scotia, and Prince Edward Island, associations were established. In the first group of provinces, the colleges were specifically delegated duties under the terms of the legislation, primarily for the protection of the public; other provincial organizations came into being for the purpose of developing scientific and other matters of purely professional interest. In the other provinces, the associations created under dental legislation elected boards or councils to carry out the terms of the Act, while the association proceeded to hold conventions to forward scientific and other matters related to the profession. Both systems have functioned well over the years, with the end effect being much the same.

With the enactment of dental legislation in Saskatchewan and Alberta, the North-West Territorial organization ceased to exist. W.D. Cowan of Regina had been the moving spirit in all its activities and continued in this capacity in Saskatchewan. He wrote a history of dentistry in the North-West Territories which was never printed in full, but a copy has become available and is the source of most of the early information respecting dentistry in the vast midwest.[5] Cowan was a man of strong convictions and forcible language, and it is said that some of his observations respecting the holders of political office of the time were cautiously deleted. The first meeting of dentists in the area had been called by Cowan in his office at Regina in July 1889. Very little space was required. Eleven dentists were named as practising then in the Territory, of whom three attended the meeting. Two or three other 'partial' dentists were named, for example: 'Dr Callendar of Toronto had taken a homestead near Regina and while his horses rested, he would occasionally insert a gold filling for a neighbour.' Decision was made to form the North-West Territorial Dental Association and Cowan was elected president, a position he held during the life of the Association and the early years of its Saskatchewan successor.[6]

Quite probably one reason for organizing at this time was that the

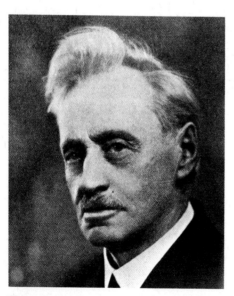

Walter Davey Cowan, DDS (1865–1934)

number of settlers was increasing at a rapid rate. Anybody could practise dentistry: no qualifications were necessary. The first objective was to secure legislation from the Territorial Council, and that body adopted an ordinance regulating the practice of dentistry in November 1889. The lawyer who drafted the legislation and piloted it through the assembly accepted as payment in full upper and lower dentures made by Cowan.

Implementation of the ordinance proved difficult, however, over a territory of almost unlimited space. Continually some individual or another began practising, often hundreds of miles away from a main centre, and the expenses of securing evidence and prosecution fell upon the few members, who were forced to pay the cost of any action out of their own pockets. The first ordinance proved faulty, and for years a continuing battle ensued to secure amendments respecting qualifications and other pertinent matters. In the meantime an influx of individuals, some qualified and some not, began practising. As president, Cowan was subject to much abuse, but in spite of it all his popularity was sustained. He was elected mayor of Regina in 1916 by an overwhelming majority and later was elected Member of Parliament. In 1903 the ordinance was amended, changing the title of the organization from Dental Association to the College of Dental Surgeons of the North-West Territories, and by 1905 there were 250 dentists registered in the Territories. However, there were not that many dentists actually practising. A number of non-residents registered simply because it was comparatively easy to do so, as good insurance for any future decision to change location during a period of rapid migration.[7]

K.C. McDonald was elected president of the British Columbia Dental Association in 1905. Later he became active politically and was elected to the British Columbia Legislature in 1916, becoming Minister of Agriculture in 1933. In the words of his daughter, 'Dentistry was my father's profession, but politics was his life.' He died in office in 1945.

Sepsis and its prevention were the most prevalent subjects of addresses and discussions at both dental and medical meetings during the early years of the present century. Beginning in the 1890s, this threat had been receiving increasing attention. Albert E. Webster of Toronto was a leader in pointing out the dangers of sepsis in the practice of dentistry.[8] He, together with others, presented methods of preventing its occurrence in many published articles. It remained for a visiting lecturer, however, to present the situation forcibly and arouse the attention of Canadian dentists.

In October 1910, William Hunter, a prominent British physician, gave an address at McGill University in which he dealt at length with sepsis, laying particular emphasis on oral sepsis and its relationship to disease. His text was published in the *Lancet*, received marked attention, was widely circulated, caused a good deal of editorial comment, and stirred great controversy among dentists for several years.[9] Seldom has any one speech had so much influence over so much time. Many of the statements in the lengthy address must have seemed radical at the time, and indeed some seem so even today. Ten years earlier, Hunter had published a paper under the title, 'Oral Sepsis as a Cause of Disease,' which had received editorial comment in professional publications including the *Dominion Dental Journal*, but had apparently attracted little more than ordinary notice. In his McGill address, later delivered at Toronto and several American cities, he claimed that he had coined the term 'oral sepsis.' To present his import fully would require almost complete quotation. In essence, he argued that oral sepsis was 'more important as a potential disease factor than any other source of sepsis in the body'; that 'if oral sepsis (and nasopharyngeal) could be successfully excluded, the other channels by which "medical sepsis" gains entrance into the body might almost be ignored'; and that 'the gums and periosteum of the sockets are the seat of numerous septic wounds.' In considerable detail he discussed the current practice of dentistry:

No one has probably had more reason than I have had to admire the sheer ingenuity and mechanical skill constantly displayed by the dental surgeon. And no one has had more reason to appreciate the ghastly tragedies of oral sepsis which his misplaced ingenuity so often carries in its train. Gold fillings, gold caps, gold bridges, gold crowns, fixed dentures, built in, on, and around diseased teeth, form a veritable mausoleum of gold over a mass of sepsis to which there is no parallel in the whole realm of medicine or surgery. The whole constitutes a perfect gold trap of sepsis of which the patient is proud and which no persuasion will induce him to part with. For has it not cost him much money, and has he not been proud to have his black roots elegantly covered with beaten gold, although no ingenuity in the world can incorporate the gold edge of the cap or crown with the underlying surfaces of the root beneath the edges of the gums? There is no rank of society free from the fatal effects on health of this surgical malpractice.

And further he stated boldly:

The medical ill-effects of this septic surgery are to be seen every day in those who are the victims of this gilded dentistry in their dirty-grey, sallow, pale, wax-like complections, and in the chronic dyspepsias, intestinal disorders, ill-health, anaemias, and nervous ('neurotic') complaints from which they suffer. In no class of patients and in no country are these, in my opinion, more common than among Americans and in America, the original home of this class of work.

Needless to say, these accusations were not accepted kindly by many in the dental profession at the time, but in the long run, together with other findings, they served to bring about a changed concept of the dentist's role. Up to this period, the preponderance of emphasis in practice had been on the side of mechanical perfection. Dental art had achieved a level of great pride for both practitioner and patient. Now the biological side of practice was forcibly presented. The teaching in dental schools had altered considerably, well ahead of Hunter, but time was required before the change would reach the operating chair. By his attack, Hunter served to hasten a process already well begun.

Looking backward, it appears a long, slow trail to the recognition of sepsis as a cause of disease. Leeuwenhoek of Holland, after inventing his microscope, reported to the Royal Society of London in 1680 that he had seen little animals running around in drops of saliva. Pasteur of France had established in 1864 the validity of the germ theory of disease, from which Lister of Great Britain had in 1865 devised the use of carbolic acid spray to exclude atmospheric germs and prevent putrefaction following surgical procedures. Koch of Germany isolated and related specific germs to specific diseases, thus creating the science of bacteriology, near the end of the nineteenth century. Others made lesser contributions along the way, but it was not until the beginning of the present century that real implementation of the sepsis theory came into practice.

As with all new theories, the reception was varied, particularly among older practitioners. Men do not leave the past lightly. Perhaps the early attitude toward sepsis is expressed better than in many explanatory words by a bit of doggerel written anonymously and printed in a number of professional journals in 1903. It is thought that the writer was an older medical practitioner.

I am somethin of a veteran jest a turnin eighty year–
A man that's hale and hearty as a stranger tew all fear;

But I've heard some news this morning, that has made
    my old head spin,
An' I'm goin', to ease my conshuns if I never speak again.
I have lived my fourscore years of life, an' never till today
Wuz I taken for a jackass or an ignorant kind of jay.
Tew be stuffed with such darned nonsense 'bout them crawlin
    bugs and worse,
That's a killin' human bein's with their microscopic germs.
They say there's microbes all about a lookin for their prey,
There's nothin' pure to eat or drink, an' no safe place to stay;
There's miasmy in the dewfall, an' malary in the sun,
Tain't safe to be outdoors at noon or when the day is done;
There's bactery in the water, an' trikeeny in the meat,
Ameeby in the atmosphere, calory in the heat;
There's corpussels an' pigments in a human bein's blood,
An' every other kind of thing, existing since the flood.
Therbacer full of nickerteen, whatever they may be –
An' yer mouth'll get all puckered by the tannin in the tea.
The butter's olymargereen, it never saw a cow;
An' things is gittin' wus from what they be just now,
Them bugs is all about us jest awaitin' for a chance
Ter navigat our vitals and tew naw us off like plants.
There's men that spend a lifetime huntin' just like a goose,
An' tackin Latin names to 'em an' lettin on 'em loose.
Now I don't believe such nonsense, an' I'm not agoin' to try
If things have come to sech a pass I'm satisfied to die,
I'll go hang me in the suller, fer I won't be sech a fool
As to wait until I'm pizened by an annymalycool.

    The most distressing phase of dental practice for both patient and dentist still was the accompanying pain. General anaesthesia, first discovered by dentists, was utilized for major operations in the mouth, but was not practical for routine work. Various preparations with a cocaine base produced local anaesthesia, but cocaine, being a potent, dangerous, and habit-forming drug, produced many untoward results in patients. In addition, this drug was associated with serious social problems.

    The first step in the development of a satisfactory local anaesthesia was the determination of the chemical structure of cocaine. After many years of study, Alfred Einhorn, a German chemist, enunciated the principle that all esters of aromatic acids produce some degree of local anaesthesia. Chemists have produced many hundreds of such esters. Procaine hydrochloride, under the proprietory name of novocain, was introduced into medical practice by Professor Braun of Germany in 1905. The first paper in English on the use of novocain in local anaesthesia was published in the *Lancet* in 1906. In 1907, novocain became available on the North American continent. The first article on it to appear in Canadian dental literature was published in the *Dominion Dental Journal* in 1908. The article stated that novocain was first used for the extirpation of a vital pulp (by pressure anaesthesia) and was considered to be less toxic than cocaine.

Due to previous experience with products of a cocaine base type, many dentists hesitated before using the new product. It was first supplied commercially in powder or tablet form, and the dentist mixed his solution as he required it. This was a cumbersome, time-consuming, and inaccurate method, and office-prepared solutions rapidly deteriorated. The idea of using commercially prepared anaesthetic solutions, as well as other drugs, in cartridges was developed by Harvey S. Cook, an American surgeon during the first world war.[10] Over the years, research has continued and improved solutions have been produced under many proprietary names. The development of satisfactory local anaesthetics brought one of the greatest assets to dental practice.

Somnoform, discovered by Rolland of Bordeaux, France, in 1901, was introduced in Canada in 1904. This anaesthetic consisted of ethyl chloride 60%; methyl hydrate 35%; and ethyl bromide 5%. Administered with comparatively simple equipment, it provided general anaesthesia of short duration. The use of somnoform became intermittently popular for a couple of decades in dental practice, and was discarded mostly because of improved local anaesthetics.

A significant event in the history of Canadian dentistry occurred in 1907 when Ashley W. Lindsay became the country's first dental missionary, sponsored by the West China Mission of the Methodist Church of Canada. A few months after receiving his dental degree from the University of Toronto, he arrived at Chengtu. No form of dental education existed in China at that time. There were a few English dentists practising, mostly in Shanghai, who employed Chinese youths on an inadequate apprenticeship basis, following which the 'students' set out to practise for themselves. By 1911, Lindsay had erected a dental hospital at Chengtu. In the meantime he was joined by John Thompson, who had graduated from the Toronto school. Gradually a Chinese dental school was developed, but staff remained a problem. Thompson died after a few years. In 1917, Lindsay was joined by Harrison Mullett, another graduate, followed by Gordon Campbell, R.N. Anderson, and Gordon Agnew. These dentists made up the staff until 1928, when three American graduates were added. At first, the Chengtu dental school was a department in the College of Medicine, and later became a College of Dentistry. In 1929, a College of Medicine and Dentistry was established by the West China Union University, with two deans. In 1937, Lindsay was appointed Vice-Chancellor of the university, a position he held until the change of regime in China in 1950, after which no foreigner could hold such a position and he was forced to leave the country. Over the years, graduates of the school had been sent to dental schools in Canada and the United States for further training. On their return, these men became members of the staff and took positions in hospitals. As a result, the school was left in 1950 with a capable Chinese staff.[11] The vision of one Canadian dentist had been accomplished.

Lindsay utilized his furlough time to pursue his own graduate education. In 1928 he obtained a Bachelor of Dental Science degree, and in 1936 his Master's degree. The University of Toronto conferred the honorary degree of Doctor of Laws on him in 1942. On his return to Canada, he was appointed editor of the *Journal of the Ontario Dental Association*, a position he held for fifteen years.

In this period also occurred another event with long-term consequences. Harold Clark was a well-respected dentist in Toronto for nearly fifty years. He had many interests, possessed a large library, and it would probably be fair to say that he was one of the more learned members of the profession in his day. In any event, his advice was sought and taken seriously. In 1906, he delivered a paper to the Ontario Dental Society on the proprietary preparations being used in dentistry, indicating that many of the dentifrices on the market were doing more harm than good. Up to this time, testing, if any was done, of proprietary preparations used within practice or by the public was haphazard. One dentist in Clark's audience, Andrew J. McDonagh, became concerned with the need for action and within a year created an organization for the purpose.

McDonagh had graduated from the Royal College of Dental Surgeons in 1887. He had engaged in general practice in Toronto for several years,

but during the early 1900s gradually limited his practice to treatment of
the tissues surrounding the teeth, being the first Canadian dentist to do so.
For several years, he had been a lecturer on pyorrhea aveolaris and a
member of the staff of the Toronto school; in 1915, what is said to be the
first chair in the world for teaching periodontology in a dental school was
established, with McDonagh as a professor. He was very active, both as a
citizen and in the interests of his profession, for his whole career.
McDonagh was a convincing clinical teacher with a keen mind devoted to
research and the advancement of periodontology at a time when this phase
of practice was at its beginning. He held many positions within the profession, and was a founding member of the American Academy of Periodontology. To him, the impossible was only something which took a little
longer to accomplish. No task for the advancement of dentistry was too
great; yet he was always ready to help another dentist with the simplest
problem.

In the day of Clark's speech, McDonagh had done some investigation into the content of dentifrices on the market and the shapes of tooth
brushes for sale. After it, he organized the Canadian Oral Prophylactic
Association with the prime purpose of developing an acceptable dentifrice
and tooth brush which dentists could recommend with impunity. The
name given the products, Hutax, was coined from two Greek words
meaning health and mouth. The motive of the new association was altruistic. The dentifrices then being sold to the public were known to contain
injurious substances and the tooth brushes were proven incapable of
accomplishing their intended purposes. Once the new products were
developed, it was initially thought, there would be no difficulty in inducing
a reputable producer to manufacture them. However, this assumption
proved incorrect, and the association itself was forced to undertake the
responsibility of manufacture. The association had a lengthy life: its
charter of incorporation was not finally surrendered until the 1940s. Yet
throughout its history, continuing difficulties occurred in finding a manufacturer who would adhere to the formula established and retain the
franchise.

In the face of commercial producers' advertising, the association depended entirely upon the recommendations of dentists. From the beginning, dentists were kept well-informed respecting its products through
their own publications and a great deal of space in the dental literature
was occupied during two decades with reports on its activities. On one
point some disagreement occurred among the leaders of the profession.

The association received a small royalty on the products, and the moneys thus received were devoted to the support of dental research and dental public health education. No other financial support was then available for either of these purposes and the need was great. However, some dentists objected to involvement in a commercial pursuit for the support of professional activities of this nature. Over the years, some sharp controversies occurred. The timing of the movement and the circumstances of the period must be taken into consideration in assessing its significance. During its existence, other agencies came into being with different methods but similar objectives, with the result that commercial products improved. But the association did its part, as well as supporting Canadian dental research and the publication of dental public health matter. The Canadian Oral Prophylactic Association was also largely responsible for making possible the creation of another organization to be treated later, the Canadian Dental Hygiene Council, which made a very substantial contribution.

The first directory of Canadian dentists was published in 1909 by the *Dominion Dental Journal*. The book in itself is a fine production in semi-hard covers, but more important it is a mine of information about the profession at this stage of its development. The book not only records the name, any degrees, and address of every Canadian dentist. It also presents the provincial dental Acts as amended to that date; the officers of all existing dental societies; the dental schools with descriptions respecting admission requirements and related matters, including the names of the complete staff and their positions in each school; manufacturers, dental laboratories, and dental supply houses; and full information on the

DENTISTS PRACTISING IN CANADA IN 1909

British Columbia	86	(350,000)
Alberta	76	(301,000)
Saskatchewan	62	(401,000)
Manitoba	93	(427,000)
Ontario	900	(2,444,000)
Quebec	231	(1,931,000)
New Brunswick	82	(346,000)
Nova Scotia	114	(483,000)
Prince Edward Island	21	(94,000)
Total	1,665	(6,777,000)

Dominion Dental Council. All was sold for a price of one dollar. Many years were to pass before another directory appeared and even then nothing so complete was attempted.

For the first time, an accurate record from the registrars of the provincial dental boards was published, showing the number of dentists practising in 1909 in Canada. (The table appears on the opposite page. The provincial population figures, in parentheses, are from the Dominion Bureau of Statistics, estimated for intercensal years.)

Some measurement of the academic qualifications of dentists then in practice is gained from the accompanying table, although the percentages given do not represent the whole picture. Many who graduated from a dental school did not bother to obtain the degree, which required another examination by the university.[12] This is particularly true of those who graduated from a Canadian school before its affiliation with a university. The age of the practising dentist was also a factor affecting the likelihood of his holding a degree. Certain observations can be safely made. Almost two-thirds of Canadian dentists possessed a degree, and the percentage was higher in the older provinces than in the new ones. The academic stature of the Canadian dentist had risen considerably in a comparatively short period.

The pages of the directory offer further opportunities to assess developments in the profession as of 1909. In spite of strenuous opposition less than a decade earlier, some thirty-six established laboratories are listed.[13] These were located mostly in the larger centres: Montreal had four, Toronto thirteen, Winnipeg four, and Vancouver two; but they also were spreading out to smaller centres such as Oshawa and Brandon. Dental supply houses were established in the main cities across the country, with eleven in Toronto alone.

Four dental schools were in operation. The Maritime Dental College at Halifax was affiliated with Dalhousie University; l'Ecole de chirurgie dentaire, de l'Université Laval was functioning at Montreal; the McGill Dental School, also at Montreal, was still a department in the Faculty of Medicine; the Royal College of Dental Surgeons at Toronto was affiliated with the University of Toronto. Later all these schools were to become faculties of the respective universities, but another two decades passed before a fifth dental school was established at the University of Alberta.[14]

By this period, the number of dental organizations had multiplied, particularly on the local level, as indicated in Appendix D. Any attempt to follow through the development of these societies would be most tedious.

Registered dentists holding doctorate degrees (DDS) practising in the year 1909

School of graduation	Province								
	B.C.	Alta.	Sask.	Man.	Ont.	Que.	N.B.	N.S.	P.E.I.
CANADA									
University of Toronto	5	17	7	24	538	3			
Bishop's College						69			
Trinity University		3			33				
McGill University			1			2			
Laval University						18			
UNITED STATES									
Philadelphia Dental College	8		2	1	11	8	7	29	
University of California	1								
Boston Dental College	1					1			
North Pacific Dental College	1								
Northwestern University	1	1	5	6	2				
Milwaukee Medical College	1		3					6	
University of Buffalo	1								1

Maryland Dental College	1						1	8	
Detroit Dental College	1	1							
Louisville College of Dental Surgery	1								
University of Pennsylvania	1	1	1	1		3	7	17	1
Chicago College of Dental Surgery	1	2	2	3	8	4			
Coll. of Physicians & Surgeons—San Francisco					1				
Baltimore College of Dental Surgery		3	1		1	4	10	24	6
Western Reserve University		2							
University of Michigan		1	1			1	1	1	
Harvard University		1	1			1	2	2	1
Denver Dental College					1	1		1	
Miami Dental College						1			
Ohio University						1			
New York Dental School						3	3	1	
Tufts Dental College							7	4	1
American College of Dental Surgery								2	
Indiana Dental College									1
Source of degree not stated	1		2	1	32	4	1		
Percentage of total number of practising dentists	30.2	39.5	43.5	38.7	69.5	53.2	47.5	83.3	52.4

SOURCE: *Canadian Dental Directory* 1909

The names or titles were altered from time to time, and of course some were not sustained. At this point in time it became the fashion to form odontological societies, all of which have disappeared or been renamed.

Progress of dental supply houses and manufacturers has been important to Canadian dentists, particularly to those pioneers who found themselves as much as two thousand miles from a source of dental supplies. By the early 1900s, advertisements are to be found for eight supply houses in Toronto, two in Montreal, and one in Halifax. Through amalgamations most of the original names of these firms have disappeared. As the West opened up, the firms in Toronto began sending agents to its larger municipalities. The first to make a trip was H.P. Temple of Toronto, in 1902. A.E. Aunger, an Alberta dentist, recalls that he received a card from a Toronto depot advising him that their agent would be at a certain hotel in Winnipeg, 800 miles away, on a certain date. If he wanted to see the agent, he had to make the trip. The establishment of western branch depots followed, first at Winnipeg in 1903, and by 1912 at other larger cities. These developments, together with greatly improved means of transportation, contributed greatly to the ability of widely scattered dentists to render services. Some of the early efforts of the dental firms seem to have been motivated more by service than profit. Today, dentists across the country find themselves with dental supplies within relatively easy reach.

Alterations in practice occurred as new products became available. In 1907 a new filling material appeared, first known as petroid cement. Originally this material, invented by Emmanuel de Trey, was produced in Zurich, Switzerland, and imported. It was easy to use, and in theory could be matched in colour to the tooth, although the early product left much to be desired in the matching of shades. By 1911 it was being manufactured on this continent under the name of synthetic porcelain, and the shades gradually improved. Like other innovations, it caused disturbances. Gold foil had stood the test of time and many dentists hesitated to substitute a product of unknown quality. The baked porcelain restoration also had come into general use and proven satisfactory. But public demand for an unnoticeable restoration at a lower fee brought the new material into increasing use.

S.W. McInnis, an outstanding leader of the profession in Manitoba, died in November 1907, at the age of 42. At the time he was president of the Canadian Dental Association. During his relatively brief career, McInnis had not only creditably occupied all possible positions the profession had to offer, but had also served as Speaker of the Manitoba Legislature, Provincial Secretary, and Minister of Education. A large number of tributes were forwarded by professional and lay organizations from across the country.

The interest of the profession in the education of the public in dental health is typified in a resolution, adopted at the 1906 meeting of the Canadian Dental Association in Montreal. It called for:[15]

1   An act requiring the periodical examination of the teeth of school children, and providing for the appointment of dentists for the purpose.
2   Revision of school books with regard to the hygiene of the mouth and teeth.
3   Distribution of suitable booklets in the public and private schools and large military camps.
4   Special instruction in this subject in normal schools.
5   Special paper on subjects of dental hygiene in examination for teacher's licence.
6   Lectures before teachers' associations and school children in public and private schools.

By the end of the period dealt with in this chapter, the beginnings of a turning-point in Canadian dentistry had been reached. The whole question of sepsis opened a new concept of dental service. Scientific programs of the future were to lay emphasis upon sterilization, the relationship of dental disease to general health, and the place of dentistry in health services. At the 1910 meeting of the Canadian Dental Association, A.E. Webster devoted the major part of his presidential address to these subjects. Of course, the trend was gradual, but the inclination to the biological concept of dentistry was definite, and continuing. It would be accelerated by other factors in the future, among them the x-ray, which was not yet in common use in practice and would not be for several years.

Often it has been said that the only thing more certain in this life than death and taxes is the inevitability of change. The degree, direction, and speed of change may vary from one period to another; but a significant feature of Canadian dentistry over the years has been that as soon as the new was proven, the profession implemented it rapidly. At this stage, with a new concept recognized, the dental schools altered their courses to meet the new environment. Dental art was not lowered, but dental science was elevated.

10

Professional freedom
1910-1914

Professional legislative freedom in Canada is unique. The first dental Act, adopted in 1868, provided that registered dentists practising in the Province of Ontario elect a board of directors to carry out the provisions of the Act in the interests of the public. This principle of freedom within the profession was copied by the other provinces with minor variation as their legislation was enacted. Some delay occurred in British Columbia, where the first Act (1886) provided for appointment of a Board by the Lieutenant-Governor in Council; in 1895, this was amended to provide for the appointment by the government of members selected from a list of ten names submitted by the British Columbia Dental Association; and in 1908 a new Act was passed, providing for the election of a Council by the qualified dentists within the province. Both the legal and medical professions had obtained this legislative freedom before dentistry.

Study of legislation in other countries indicates that the established methods of governing the professions and their services fall into two main categories. In the first, appointments are made to a governing board or council by the government of the day, either wholly or in part, sometimes from a list of names submitted by the representative professional organization and sometimes not. Where the government does not make all the appointments, it usually controls the majority of appointments and the profession, generally by election, a minority. In the second category of legislation, the governing of professional services is entirely under the control of a department or division of the government.

On only two occasions has the system been seriously questioned in Canada. As a result of charges that the professions were abusing their privileges, the Ontario Government set up a commission of enquiry which reported in 1918. It absolved the professions, with a few recommendations for improving the system. In 1947, the Saskatchewan Government threatened to take over the administration of the professions: considerable public controversy resulted, and in the end the government withdrew. Accusations against the right of self-government by the professions appear from time to time, generally on isolated points, often bizarre, and far from the fact when investigated. Often the public does not recognize that the professions, through the legislation, are accountable for their actions to the legislatures. They have not thirsted for the ichor of power, but rather have sought to provide services of quality in the best possible manner. In carrying out this aim, criticism from within the profession has often been more severe than that from the laity. Much of the progress made by the health professions in Canada is credited to the fact of self-government.[1]

Reference was made earlier to the outcry that arose from some dentists that too many graduates would be produced following the construction of a larger school at Toronto in 1896. By 1902, it was already necessary to increase the size of that building by approximately fifty per cent. This need came about for three main reasons. First, it had been announced that the course would be increased from three years to four years in 1903, which automatically increased the number of applications before the extension took place. Second, a public demand existed in Ontario for more graduates. Third, no school existed in Canada west of Toronto, and an increasing number of students were applying for admission from the West. This situation was to exist for the next twenty years, and at times a high percentage of students at Toronto came from outside Ontario. As the years passed, a similar situation developed at McGill, and to a lesser extent at Dalhousie.

In 1907, the Hospital Trust notified the Ontario Dental Board that they desired to purchase the property occupied by the dental school in order to expand the Toronto General Hospital. This created a situation somewhat similar to that of 1896, when the school now threatened was built. In order to obtain the secure backing of the profession, the Board circulated a questionaire to all Ontario dentists, outlining the situation and specifically calling for a vote on seeking establishment of the school as a faculty of the University of Toronto. Ninety-five per cent of the ballots returned were favourable. Several meetings were held between representatives of the Board and the university. The university did not raise any substantial objections to establishment of a dental faculty, but stated it was impossible to do so in the forseeable future for financial reasons. Once more the profession rose to an emergency, and proceeded to purchase property at the corner of College and Huron Streets: a much larger school was erected, and equipped in the most modern style, without any financial assistance from outside the profession. In the course of only a few years, even this building, which was considered at the time fully adequate, had to be enlarged.

To a considerable extent, the building experience of the Toronto school reflects the rapid expansion of dental service during the early part of the twentieth century in Canada. The other three schools made adjustments during the same period. The Laval school moved in 1913 to the new Laval dental hospital in Montreal's Latin Quarter, and in the next year a new dental clinic was established by McGill at the Montreal General Hospital. A dental faculty had already been established at Dalhousie University in 1912.

With the expansion of the schools came the need for full-time staff. No longer could a school be administered by a man who at the same time was conducting a busy practice. A.W. Thornton, a staff member of the Toronto school, was appointed full-time head of the McGill school in 1913. Eudore Dubeau was a full-time dean of the Laval school, and the Royal College of Dental Surgeons at Toronto increased its number of full-time men, including A.E. Webster. Dalhousie, with a smaller number of students, was able to carry on with a part-time staff until much later. For the leaders in dental education during this period, notable contributions often involved a real sacrifice in time away from lucrative practices. While service on a teaching staff might hold considerable honour, the recompense, if any, was insignificant. The acceptance of a full-time position on a teaching staff meant diminished income.

Eudore Dubeau was born at Quebec City in 1875. After attendance at Saint Mary's Jesuit College, he obtained his Arts degree at l'Université Laval in 1892 and his dental degree from Bishop's College in 1895. Almost immediately after graduation, he was recognized for his ability and appointed secretary of the Quebec Dental Board, a position he held from 1900 to 1923. He was a founding member of the Canadian Dental Association and served as its president from 1904 to 1906. With the founding of the Laval dental school in 1905, he became its first dean, and continued in that position when in 1920 the school became the Faculté de chirurgie dentaire, Université de Montréal. He retired in 1945. Dr

Dubeau was the first Canadian dentist to take an active interest in the International Dental Federation, attending the first session in 1900 in Paris, France, and receiving at that time a medal as a founding member. Outside his profession he was also active; he was Consul in Montreal for Portugal, and a member of Montreal City Council. During his career, the French Republic bestowed several decorations on him, including those of Officer d'Academie (1909), Officer d'Instruction Publique (1916), and Chevalier d'Instruction d'honneur (1923). He also received the award of Honneur et Merite (Haiti) in 1935 and was made Chevalier of the Order of Christ (Portugal) in 1936. He died in 1953.

A.W. Thornton was a dentist of exceptional ability. He was born at Perth, Ontario, and taught school for twelve years before studying dentistry. After receiving his degree from the University of Toronto in 1890, he practised in western Ontario for twelve years, during which he inspired the organization of the Western Ontario Dental Society. In 1903, he moved to Toronto to take a position on the staff of the Toronto school. Ten years later he was appointed head of the McGill school. In large part he is credited with the establishment of dentistry as a full Faculty at McGill, which occurred in 1920. Thornton continued as dean until 1927,

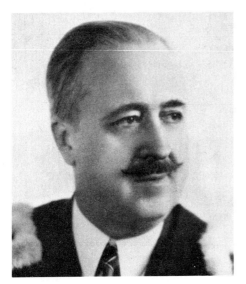

Eudore Dubeau, BSC, DDS, Doyen, Faculté de chirurgie dentaire, Université de Montréal, 1905–44

when failing health forced him to retire. He served as president of the
American Association of Dental Schools in 1926–7. He was a literary
man, a poet of no mean calibre, and a very popular after-dinner speaker.
His ability in this direction did much to initiate the public of Quebec in
dental education. He died in 1931, aged 73.

The name of Willmott and Ontario dentistry were synonymous for
half a century. J.B. Willmott died in June 1915 at seventy-eight years of
age, still in office as dean of the Royal College of Dental Surgeons and
secretary of the Ontario Dental Board. At his death, glowing tributes were
paid to him in the lay press and in resolutions spread on the minutes
of dental organizations, large and small, across the country. He was a
recognized builder of the profession, particularly in the area of dental
education, which he recognized as its cornerstone. To a large extent
through his energy and far-sighted views, dentistry had been elevated
from a motley crowd of expert technicians to a profession of recognized
academic standing. Often he was misjudged, but any man who succeeds
in satisfying everybody can be sure that his work will not endure. He had
to face many difficulties and some of the prejudices which meet every
pioneer, but so many firsts occurred at his instigation that it would be

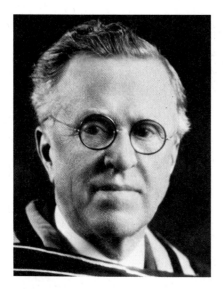

A.W. Thornton, DDS, Dean of the
Faculty of Dentistry, McGill University, 1913–27

almost impossible to compose a complete list. He was honoured by the profession on many occasions. In 1910, when the new Toronto school was built, the profession, by individual contribution, installed a large stained glass commemorative window in his honour, which was carefully transferred when the present home of the Faculty of Dentistry was built during the 1950s. In 1914, the University of Toronto conferred the honorary degree of Doctor of Laws upon him, the first Canadian dentist so honoured.[2] In later life he had difficulties in dealing with the rising dental generation, but there is nothing unusual in this situation. Devoted to his profession, he was pertinacious, resourceful, and ingenious in advancing it throughout his long life.

His son, Walter E. Willmott, succeeded him as secretary of the Ontario Dental Board, and held the position for twenty-five years. Walter Willmott graduated from the Royal College of Dental Surgeons in 1888. The following year he graduated from the Philadelphia Dental College, and immediately was appointed the first full-time staff member of the Toronto school. Over a period of forty years on the staff, he taught nearly every subject on the curriculum, and at the same time served in some administrative capacity or other in the school. Early in the 1930s, he

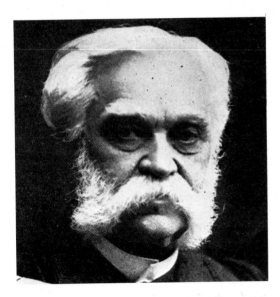

James Branston Willmott, DDS, MDS, LLD, Dean of the Royal College of Dental Surgeons, 1875–1915

severed his direct connection with the school and became full-time secretary of the Dental Board. Up to his death in 1951 he was greatly respected by the profession at large and received many honours.

In the previous chapter, the other giant of Canadian dental education during this period, Frank Woodbury of Dalhousie, was introduced. Of course, the accomplishments of these men were attained only through the assistance and co-operation of a host of colleagues in the schools. From the length of faithful and effective service as a staff member Frederick G. Henry stands forth prominently in the lists. He was born in Montreal in 1870. Before studying dentistry, he spent ten years in commercial life, which undoubtedly contributed to his ability to understand his fellow man. Immediately following graduation in dentistry from Bishop's College in 1899, he began his teaching career on the staff of that school. When it was taken over by McGill (a move in which he played an important part), Henry continued as a member of the staff, and assisted in the change from departmental to faculty status in 1920. During the earlier years he taught materia medica and pathology, also serving in numerous capacities. He reached retirement age in 1935, but there was no one to take his place and he served on for a time. In 1935, he was appointed professor emeritus. In 1914, McGill University conferred on him the DDS degree (ad eundem). He was 94 when he died in 1964. These bare facts do not represent his greatest contribution. He was greatly respected and loved by students who sought his counsel on all occasions, and during his latter years this was his main service. Unassuming in character, quiet in manner, highly principled, he was a maker of professional men.

None of these leaders in dental education found the task easy. A constant flow of obstacles arose, difficult to overcome. One typically frustrating incident occurred at McGill. By custom on this continent, graduates in dentistry have received the degree of Doctor of Dental Surgery. No question arose at any other Canadian university in this respect. McGill, however, first granted only a degree of Graduate in Dental Surgery. In 1908 it decided to grant the degree of Doctor of Dental Surgery, and so stated in the calendar for that year; but when the certificate was issued it read, *Doctoris in Arts Dentalis Scientia*. This caused further controversy. It was not until 1918 that Thornton was able to obtain the desired certificate for the degree.

As in the other professions, the idea of indentureship training had a slow demise. During the early days, when formal courses were of short duration, ample reason existed for apprenticeship training; but as the academic courses increased in length, the need for it diminished. However, indentureship had been an established custom from the beginning and practising dentists strongly protested against any change. By the end of the 1890s, leaders of the profession were advocating shortening the period and in some cases doing away with it entirely. Perhaps the system should be explained. In those days a student intending to study dentistry could not simply apply to a school. First he had to find a dentist who was willing to sign an indentureship contract with him, and who was also acceptable to the dental board of the province. During his indentureship, the student was required to attend the established courses of instruction at an acceptable dental school. From time to time, the periods of indentureship and academic courses altered. By 1900 the term of indentureship was four complete calendar years, during which the apprentice was required to attend a recognized dental school for three sessions of approximately five months each. In 1903, the academic course was increased to four sessions and indentureship remained the same. The training period was measured in calendar years, not the academic years of today.

The pros and cons of indentureship occupy much space in Canadian dental literature during the early years of the present century. Many dentists took a pragmatic position – that the schools taught theory but a real dentist was produced through practical experience in the office. Educators and members of the dental boards, through experience, possessed the opposite view. To them, indentureship was filled with abuse and uncontrollable; the student in the dental office learned questionable methods, often contradicting teaching in the school, and on many occasions was left without proper supervision. In 1908, action was taken in Ontario to end dental education by preceptor. However, the feeling was so strong that a student could not be trained in a dental school to operate a practice, that indentureship with a practitioner remained compulsory during the summer preceding final year. In 1911, students in Ontario were granted a choice, of attending a summer session at the dental school or indenturing with a practitioner, and in 1912 compulsory indentureship was abolished entirely. In the other provinces, indentureship gradually disappeared during the following decade, except on a voluntary basis.

Directly related to the disappearance of indentureship, there occurred several alterations in the methods of practice. One did not cause the other, but each was reinforced by the other. Until well after the turn of the century, it was believed that everything even remotely connected with the practice of dentistry must be performed by a licensed dentist himself or by a registered dental student under his direct supervision. The dental boards attempted to enforce this concept, and many dentists were disciplined for employing other personnel in any capacity. As noted earlier attempts to establish laboratories were harshly dealt with. The laboratory was a most important component of the dental office, and it was there that indentured students spent most of their time. The birth pains that introduced auxiliary personnel into dentistry were long and severe. Yet in spite of prohibitions, the number of outside dental laboratories increased, and dentists employed technicians other than registered dental students. Initially, and with extremely few exceptions, the persons so employed were male. As dental laboratories became established, however, the need for such personnel in the office lessened. Women began to be hired in increasing numbers for duties other than purely mechanical. By 1910, although many dentists still performed the whole service for the patient in their own offices, laboratories were established across the country. A dental editorial in 1914 stated that, 'It is in the interest of the public from an economic standpoint that every person shall perform the highest service that he is capable of. It is waste of money to educate a dental surgeon and have him spend his time performing operations that might be done by a nurse, an assistant or dental mechanic.'[3] The greatest overall factor contributing to this process was the changing concept of dental service. As emphasis shifted from mechanical to biological, the fabrication of appliances became incidental. And so did the reliance on cheap, indentured labour to do that work.

In 1910, the last great land rush got underway. The Peace River country, approximately 120,000 square miles with over a million acres of fine arable land, straddles the northern border of British Columbia and Alberta. The area had been well-known by fur traders (Fort Dunvegan, a fur trading post, was built in 1815) and by gold seekers, but its great agriculture potential was not recognized until the end of the first decade of the present century. Transportation was the difficult problem. Edmonton was the jumping-off place, but owing to an enormous muskeg area between it and the Peace River country, summer travel had to be by river and lake. The faith of the early settlers has been amply rewarded. The visitor today finds prosperous towns supported by the physical riches of good black soil, gas, oil, coal, water power, timber, and pulp wood.

The first dentist arrived in the Peace River country in March 1911.

Albert Sproule was born near Parrsboro, Nova Scotia, in 1869. His older son, J.C. Sproule, a noted geologist of Calgary, has provided details of his adventures.[4] The story pertains not only to the history of Canadian dentistry, but also to the lives of settlers moving from one of the oldest settled areas of Canada to its newest frontier. Albert Sproule was an only son with ten sisters. He remained on the family farm, helping his father educate the sisters, until he was twenty-six years old. Then, with practically no education himself, he went to Boston, where by intensive study he covered the preliminary academic requirements in one year and gained admission to the Boston Dental College. He graduated in 1898. After a short interval he returned to Parrsboro, where he practised some twelve years. During this time he helped his father pay off the debts incurred in educating his sisters – in accordance with the tradition of Nova Scotia, where education has always held a top priority.

People who knew Sproule personally have described how he was seized with the idea of serving where the need was greatest. As news of the Peace River country spread rapidly across Canada in the winter of 1910–11, he decided to go there. By this time he was married and had two sons, the youngest only one year old. With his family, Sproule travelled by train to Edmonton and then to Edson, a station some 150 miles further west. From here nothing more than a trail existed to his destination of Grande Prairie, approximately 200 miles to the northwest. In a caboose which he built himself, carried on sleighs and drawn by two teams of horses, the family reached Grande Prairie in early 1911. An inventory of his equipment and supplies, if it were available, would make interesting reading. Sproule had no illusions about where he was going and realized that he would probably find it necessary to farm, at least part of the time, in the new territory. He did actually take up land. However, people came from such great distances and in such great numbers for dental service that after a few years he found himself subsidizing the operation of the farm from his professional fees. He therefore gave up agriculture. To meet the requests from distant points all over the Peace River country, he designed a portable dental office, probably the first in Canada, and during the summer months visited outlying settlements. One of his student assistants on these northern treks was a young man named Hector MacLean, later dean of Dentistry at the University of Alberta.

Sproule was a perfectionist, not only in dentistry, but in all else he attempted to do. He was an inventor and spent his latter years working on patents for gas furnaces and gas appliances, now widely used. Another of his patents had to do with house-trailers, a by-product of his portable dental office and the caboose he had built in 1911. He died in April 1941. A pioneer neighbour of Dr Sproule in Grande Prairie wrote to me: 'The doctor was quite a colourful figure in the early days of Grande Prairie, holding many public positions of authority and his wife was a lovely singer and played the piano beautifully.' He also recalled that 'on the trail, the doctor was known as an aristocrat, by reason of the fact that he drove horses instead of oxen, which were the predominant mode of power.'[5]

In spite of its importance, professional journalism has always been beset with difficulties. From its introduction in 1889, the monthly *Dominion Dental Journal* was the only dental journal in Canada. It depended entirely upon individual subscriptions for support, and considerable disparity existed between the number of subscribers and the total number of dentists in the country. While dental organizations recognized the journal as an official organ, none contributed to its support. During this period, Wallace Seccombe conceived the idea of publishing a new dental journal, supported by advertising, and mailed free to every Canadian dentist each month. Seccombe was a most energetic dentist who possessed as well considerable business ability. His endeavour, *Oral Health*, was born in 1911. He continued as both publisher and editor until his death in 1936. While the format has been altered from time to time, this journal has continued to be published to the present.

Activities in the field of dental public education continued during the 1910s. Initially, great faith was placed in action by government. Year after year, dental organizations submitted resolutions or briefs to governments, pointing out the existing oral health of Canadian children and emphasizing the need for action. No department of health then existed in any Canadian government. Provincial boards of health did exist, but their budgets were minimal. A historic cairn on the grounds of the Parliament Buildings at Fredericton records the fact that the first Ministry of Health in the British Empire was established by the New Brunswick Government in 1918. The plaque reads in part, 'the resulting benefits were so noticeable that the example was followed in other parts of Canada and the Empire.' However, it was another decade before all Canadian governments established such departments. As a consequence, since the emphasis was on children, submissions in this period were directed to the Departments of Education. As noted previously, permissive legislation had been obtained for dental inspection of school children in two provinces, but the responsibility for this rested with local school boards, who did not always accept the need.

By 1910, a definite change of attitude had occurred within the profession. Faith in government action had diminished and it was realized that the profession would have to provide the leadership. Men like J.G. Adams of Ontario and George Kerr Thompson of Nova Scotia had been aware of this for years, but it took time for the rank and file of the dentists to realize it. When they did, active educational committees, as they were named at this period, were set up by most dental organizations across Canada.

Through the energetic leadership of Wallace Seccombe, with R.J. Reade as secretary, the educational committee of the Ontario Dental Society rapidly developed an amazing list of accomplishments. It produced booklets and, through the Department of Agriculture, arranged for publication and distribution of copies in enormous quantities at government expense. Lectures on dental health were organized for nurses in hospitals and teachers' training schools. The appointment of a dental inspector, W.D. Doherty, for the Toronto schools was secured. (It is notable that the stated purpose of his appointment was to prevent decay of teeth, rather than to inspect teeth when decayed.) Charts and exhibits were prepared for use in the schools. Dental clinics were established at the Toronto General Hospital and the Hospital for Sick Children in 1911. A free dental clinic for the poor children of Toronto was launched in 1913, in the charge of J.A. Bothwell under the Medical Health Officer; this was the first recognition by a Canadian municipality of its responsibility in the treatment of dental diseases.[6] While such activities became commonplace later, they were new at the time. The results were rapidly apparent and the endeavours copied in the other provinces. While the work of these committees on education was directed toward the public, within the profession they served to re-orient thinking and establish a strong attitude toward the prevention of dental diseases.

Wallace Seccombe was a leader of great energy and ability. Up to the time of his activity in the area of education of the public, efforts had been largely confined to the repair of damage in the mouths of children. In the main, he deserves the credit for the alteration of emphasis to preventing the damage before it occurred. He was responsible for initiating the movement toward prevention, which has since continued, with increased emphasis, in Canadian dentistry. In 1915, he established what is said to be the first chair of preventive dentistry in any dental school. Like other strong leaders, his activities did not always endear him to his confreres, largely because he was not content to wait for everyone to be converted to the obviously right procedure. Many 'cut and thrust' arguments arose, but Seccombe won in the end. One humorous incident occurred at the annual meeting of the Ontario Dental Society. Seccombe was opposed to the activities of the Canadian Oral Prophylactic Association in the field of dental health education, and Andrew J. McDonagh was president of that organization. Seccombe had pointed out at length the iniquities of selling the public a product in order to educate them. With Irish wit, McDonagh arose and said: 'Well, boys, you know Wallace and I have these little arguments at meetings and after the meeting is over, we go out and get gloriously drunk together,' and sat down. Everyone in the audience knew that Seccombe was a teetotaler – and that McDonagh drank sparingly if at all.

Owing to the small number of dentists in Nova Scotia, New Brunswick, and Prince Edward Island, efforts were made to hold combined meetings. The first was held at Digby in 1898, and was successful. Owing to the guarding of provincial rights, however, any permanent organization was steadfastly avoided, and officers were elected for the current meeting only. Such interprovincial meetings were held at irregular intervals at first, but gradually developed into the Atlantic Provinces Dental Association with regular conventions.

The British Columbia Dental Society meanwhile became inactive. In the 1890s it had held annual meetings with programs that are surprisingly modern. By 1908, however, the society wavered, probably in part because of the alterations in legislation related at the beginning of this chapter. The Act of 1908 created the College of Dental Surgeons of British Columbia and provided for the election of a council by the members of the College. The date of this new legislation and the diminished activity by the Society coincide. The new council largely took over the control of activities related to the profession. However, a skeleton society remained in existence. At a reorganization meeting in 1916, W.J. Lea was elected president, with J.E. Black as retiring president; and since then annual meetings have been held regularly. In 1920, the name was changed from Society to Association.

The first mention of the term 'state medicine' to be found in Canadian dental literature occurred in 1911, when a joint meeting was called of the Toronto Academy of Medicine and the Ontario Dental Society to discuss the subject.[7] The news media of that time were carrying many items about the introduction of a national insurance plan by the British Parliament over the objections of the health professions.[8] The subject was to absorb the attention of the health professions in Canada at a much later date.

By 1914, the profession was well organized throughout the whole country. Each province, though the nature was varied, had satisfactory dental organizations which have remained much the same to the present day. Local societies, first in the larger centres and then in other areas, had come into being. Coincidentally came a strengthening of the voice of the profession and increased public education in dental health.

11
War years (I)
1915-1919

As a nation, Canada has been involved in three major wars which occurred with intervals of roughly twenty years – the South African war, the
first world war, and the second world war. Full-scale war has always
instigated rapid change within the countries involved, including the development of their professions. Canadian dentistry is no exception: its
history might be written in parts divided by war.

The beginnings of Canadian military dentistry in the South African
war have already been described. From the first two dentists sent overseas
in 1900 it was a long way, however, to the establishment of an effective
dental corps. Much of the initial credit must go to the persistent efforts
of Ira Bower and to the interest of the Canadian Dental Association, which
took up the question of dental care for military personnel at its founding
meeting in 1902. The proceedings of the Association record a progressive
effort at every meeting over the next four decades to establish an efficient
corps, which would be independent but with ranks and pay commensurate
with that of the medical corps. On many subjects, the Association found
difficulty in securing harmonious internal agreement, but on this objective
there was complete unanimity, with ardent support by all the dental
organizations across Canada.

After several interviews with authorities, a General Order was passed
in July 1904 which reorganized the Army Medical Services into two
separate branches, the Army Medical Department and the Regimental
Medical Service. The former consisted of the Medical Staff and the Army
Medical Corps. The latter consisted of the Permanent Active Medical
Corps and the Militia Army Medical Corps, comprising medical officers,

dental surgeons, and nursing sisters. On appointment, dental surgeons were given the relative rank of lieutenant, and after five years' service that of captain, but it was provided that in no case was the official designation to be other than Dental Surgeon. On organization, the number of dental surgeons was to be eighteen. The first dentist whose appointment was gazetted, on 10 September 1904, was W.T. Hackett of Oakville, Ontario.

This initial General Order contained an anomaly. Although the dental surgeons were to be part of the Militia Army Medical Corps, the order specifically referred to the establishment of a 'Dental Corps.' This wording may have come through the intensive efforts of the committee representing the profession; the actuality was far from their true objective of an independent body. The order's importance lies in the fact that, for the first time, dental surgeons were recognized as an essential part of the military establishment.

This early progress resulted from the experience of the South African war. But Canada is not a military nation. Her history between wars is one of dispersion and reduction of military units. Nevertheless, the committee representing the profession continued their efforts and gradually made gains. Qualifications for military appointment were established. The initial equipment provided by the Army was rudimentary, and some improvements were obtained. The type of service rendered was elementary, and some betterment was gained. The length of service before promotion from lieutenant to captain was reduced from five years to three. In 1908, during the annual meeting of the Canadian Dental Association at Ottawa, the first meeting of the Army Dental Service was held. Two years later the establishment was increased to twenty-six dental surgeons – the service was proving itself. Yet there was still much left to achieve. Certain matters rankled – among them, the fact that the promoted dental surgeon was designated 'honorary' captain and no provision was made for any higher rank. In negotiations with the government, the appointed representatives of the profession were in the main Bowers of Ottawa, J.M. Magee of Saint John, and George Kerr Thompson of Halifax. During an interview in 1912, the Minister of Militia stated that 'Canada was now doing more in respect to dental services than any other country in the world.' At the same interview the Minister requested that the Canadian Dental Association present an outline of a scheme for the establishment of a dental corps directly to him, rather than through the usual channels. This was done in keeping with the Association's adopted policy.

This then was the situation when, in August 1914, war was declared which would involve over 600,000 Canadians during the next four years. Initially, the dental requirement for recruits was 'that the candidates' teeth are to be in good order and the loss or decay of 10 teeth will be considered a disqualification'; artificial teeth were 'not recognized.' Very rapidly, recruits came forth. When the first Canadian contingent of 33,000 men sailed overseas, ten sets of dental equipment accompanied them. Yet in spite of all that had been attempted, the examination and care of soldiers' teeth was still chaotic. The dentists who had been attached to the militia for a good number of years had never been more than a kind of fifth wheel. Recruits were examined for oral health by physicians and even drill sergeants. Men were rejected whose teeth were actually in very good condition, and many were accepted whose mouths were a constant source of danger. Many received no physical examination of any kind. Soon requests arrived from England for dental units to be established at base hospitals. The few dentists in the militia were in no position to cope with the numbers involved, and there was little inducement for private practitioners to join as dental surgeons under the service conditions. On a voluntary basis, civilian dentists organized themselves to examine applicants at recruitment centres and their services were gladly accepted by commanding officers.[1]

The call for dental services at base hospitals brought an early response from McGill, which thus became the first university to offer a medical unit for overseas service. The unit was entitled No 3 Canadian General Hospital (McGill), and was organized entirely within the university. This unit consisted of 35 officers, 75 nurses, and 224 other ranks. Among the officers were two dentists, Captain G.H.A. Stevenson, who appears in the listing as Officer in charge of Dentistry, and Captain L.H. Thornton, the son of the dean.[2] The other ranks were made up of students, many of them registered in Medicine and Dentistry. Among them was Earl M. Laurin, then in his second year, and later a prominent Montreal dentist. The men arrived in England in May 1915, refused to be split, and were established as a unit in France on 14 June 1915. A dental clinic was immediately established, the first, as far as Canadian dentistry is concerned, to operate in a field of military action. The most famous member of this unit undoubtedly was Lieutenant-Colonel John McCrae, who was in charge of medicine and second in command. He died of pneumonia in France shortly after writing 'In Flanders Fields,' a poem which has obtained a lasting place in modern anthologies.[3] Queen's University organized a medical unit soon after McGill, taking on its strength Captain E.B. Sparks, who practised dentistry at Kingston for many years.

The first military dental clinic in Canada was opened in March 1915 at the Canadian National Exhibition grounds at Toronto. Permission had been granted by the Minister of Militia, General Sir Sam Hughes, who showed great interest in the clinic and made an official inspection. Shortly after, he announced unofficially that he had authorized the formation of a separate Dental Corps and appointed J. Alex Armstrong, an Ottawa dentist, as Director of Dental Services, with the rank of colonel. Undoubtedly, this action took place as a result of pressure from both commanding officers of the militia and the activities of dental organizations across the country. Actually, Armstrong was gazetted as a lieutenant-colonel, on 2 April 1915, and began his duties immediately in organizing The Canadian Army Dental Corps.

Up to this date, eighty-two dentists had joined the forces as dental surgeons with the honorary rank of lieutenant, and they became the nucleus of the newly formed Corps. Other dentists who had been active in

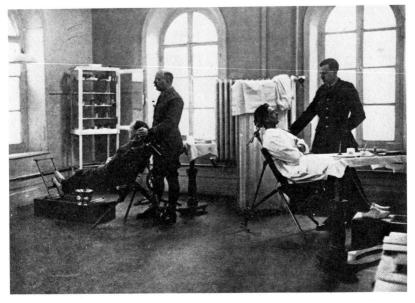

Military dentistry in France during the first world war. The dentists are G.H.A. Stevenson (*left*) and L.H. Thornton. The site is a Jesuit college at Boulogne

the militia were in service but not as dentists in their respective military units, generally with higher ranks than those serving in the Corps, and for the most part they continued to serve with these units throughout the war. Once the Corps was established, the enlistment of dentists increased rapidly.

Details from the military viewpoint have been related elsewhere.[4] The intention here is to portray more particularly developments as they affected the dental profession as a whole. On 24 June 1915, the first contingent of the Corps left Montreal. It consisted of 151 men, of whom fifty-three were graduate dentists and the others were either undergraduates or experienced laboratory men with the rank of sergeant. On arrival in England, clinic and laboratory headquarters were established at Shorncliffe, and the dental service went into operation. The demand was even greater than anticipated and very quickly a call for more men arose. Before the war

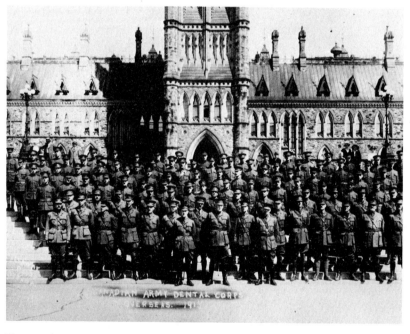

First contingent of the Canadian Army Dental Corps overseas, 1915

was over, nearly one-quarter of all Canadian graduate dentists were members of the Corps, and an undetermined number of other dentists were serving with other units.

Many problems arose in supplying the necessary personnel. The dental schools accelerated classes, and entire graduating classes went directly into the Corps. The demand for dental sergeants (assistants) became urgent, and the Toronto school generously placed equipment and staff at the disposal of the military for training. Civilian dental service was denuded in many rural areas and greatly reduced in urban areas. The public accepted this as a condition of war, an attitude which was somewhat different during the second world war. One or two incidents occurred during this period, however, that were occasions for professional alarm. In the dying hours of the Saskatchewan Legislature in 1916, an amendment to the Dental Act was passed under which a dentist who had a licence to practise could employ a man who was not a dentist to practise under the dentist's name, though he travelled from town to town throughout the province. The Saskatchewan College of Dental Surgeons had no knowledge of the amendment until after the close of the session. A few weeks later a patient died in the chair of one of these unqualified practitioners, causing a public uproar. The amendment was short-lived. A somewhat similar action that occurred in Nova Scotia is described in the next chapter.

The kind of dental service best suited for men in the forces became a subject of considerable discussion. Initially the policy of the military authorities was to perform necessary services to last two years, but as the war lengthened their attitude changed. The number of applicants rejected for dental reasons soon brought about the addition to the services of vulcanite dentures, which had not been permitted at the beginning. Military dental service gradually settled down principally to extractions, vulcanite dentures, amalgam, and oxy-phosphate fillings. While it was a primitive kind of dentistry, it had the merit of clearing the mouth of infection and restoring efficiency of mastication. And some significant advances were made.

From almost the beginning of the war, a disease which became known as 'trench mouth' was one of the main problems facing the Dental Corps. This acute stomatitis incapacitated large numbers of soldiers. Its clinical history was fairly well recorded, but the pathology was unknown. The Corps organized a special study and devised a method of treatment which controlled the disease. Another notable area of treatment was in maxillofacial cases, that brought together surgeons and dentists in unprecedented achievements. The use of the x-ray, the introduction of new dental techniques, and the development of numerous instruments and appliances, were all accelerated in meeting wartime emergencies.

Several subsidiary efforts contributed greatly to the success of the Corps. While the government supplied instruments and materials, there was no provision for numerous other essentials. To meet this need, an Army Dental Fund was established and members of the profession and the public contributed. Wives of dentists formed auxiliaries which kept up a generous flow of parcels containing hand-knitted socks and sweaters, food, and cigarettes to dentists overseas.

By 1917, the dental service regulations called for a Director-General of Dental Services with the rank of full colonel, six lieutenant-colonels, and other officers. The establishment called for one dental surgeon to every five hundred men in the services. The *Canadian Gazette*, in London, England, testified to the success in a report that 'the Canadian Army was the only army in the world, that attempted to send its soldiers to the front dentally fit. To Canada, belongs the honour of being the first country in the world to organize and put a separate dental corps in the field; and New Zealand's Army is the only other one that has another such corps, though it is understood that the Americans are organizing a dental corps. In all the other armies, the dental corps is part of the medical corps.'[5]

Two main points were causing the representatives of the profession concern, however. The first was that the Corps was established on a wartime basis only; its future became an issue on which a number of presentations were made. One of the early actions taken by the Union Government after it took office in Ottawa late in 1917 was to make the Corps a permanent part of the army. The Canadian profession read this announcement with pride. The other matter of concern was the independence of the Corps, a status the profession had pressed for from the beginning in 1902. The permanent establishment applied to service in Canada only. The Minister of Militia had stated repeatedly from the first that the Dental Corps was independent, but there appeared to be strong opposition among the military authorities. In Canada, where the communications were direct from the Corps to the Adjutant-General, there was no, or little, difficulty respecting this matter, but the situation altered overseas. In England, the point was controversial throughout the war and Canadian dentists serving soldiers in France were drafted into the Army Medical Corps.

On both these matters, the battle had to be fought again at the beginning of the second world war. Between 1918 and 1939, economy-minded governments all but wiped out many of the establishments of the first world war, including the Dental Corps. As will be seen later, however, such action did not deter the profession in its endeavours to establish the Corps on a satisfactory basis in readiness for any future catastrophe.

Following the war, demobilization brought a new set of problems. On discharge, every man was supposed to be given medical and dental examinations. If further dental treatment was found necessary, which was the case with the vast majority, the discharged soldier was given a certificate entitling him to the treatment prescribed at public expense. Theoretically, this arrangement seemed good. But at some demobilization centres, despite valiant efforts by the members of the Corps, there were just not sufficient personnel to provide adequate examinations in the rush out of the forces. In addition, dentists in the Corps were themselves anxious for discharge in order to re-establish civilian practice. Other troubles arose when the federal Department of Soldiers' Civil Re-establishment issued regulations in respect to dental services for returned soldiers, with a fee schedule attached. Immediate protest occurred within the profession, mainly on two points. First, the fee schedule was criticized, both for its limitation of services and for the fees allowed. Second, the administration of the plan was attacked because it was to be entirely by medical personnel. A journal editorial stated, 'It is difficult to understand how the self-respecting dentist in civil practice, could submit to having an officer who knows nothing about dentistry dictate to him what dental operations are to be done and what is to be paid for them.'[6] As a result of the protest, the department appointed a director of dental services. With adjustments from time to time, this arrangement was to remain in force until after the second world war.

Among those dentists who served during the war in units other than the Dental Corps, John S. Stewart of Lethbridge, born in 1877 and still enjoying an active life as this was written, is one of the more notable. His life encompasses practically the entire development period of western Canada. His family moved from Ontario to the North-West Territories, in the area that became Alberta, when he was a youngster. For a short period, he taught school. In 1899, he joined the Strathcona Horse as a private and served in the South African war where he won the Queen's medal with bars for bravery. On his return he gained admission to the Royal College of Dental Surgeons at Toronto, graduating and obtaining his dental degree from Trinity in 1903. In the same year he began practice at Lethbridge, Alberta, where he remained in practice until his retirement in 1960, with the exception of time spent in military service. To improve his army qualifications, he attended the Royal Military College at Kingston during 1907–8, graduating with the rank of major. In 1911, he was elected to the Legislative Assembly of Alberta, where he served for fourteen years. On the outbreak of hostilities in 1914, he joined the Canadian Expeditionary Forces, was promoted to lieutenant-colonel, and went overseas in command of the Seventh Artillery Brigade. In 1917 he was promoted to brigadier general in command of the Third Division, Canadian Artillery and led his division through all the engagements in which the Canadian Corps participated, being wounded twice. He received many awards, including the Distinguished Service Order, Companion of the Order of St. Michael and St. George, and Croix de Guerre. In 1930 he was elected to the House of Commons and served there for four years. In the midst of all his activities, he continued to conduct a highly ethical practice in his city and took a prominent, but unassuming, part in community affairs. The city of Lethbridge recognized him on many occasions, including the naming in 1956 of General Stewart School. The University of Alberta conferred the honorary degree of Doctor of Laws on him in 1957. The ardent spirit of this remarkable Canadian at ninety years of age is represented in a private communication to the author, written in fine legible longhand which begins: 'Yours of the 28th came this A.M. and as I have finished the chores, swept the garage, shovelled the snow, even on the boulevard, therefore with a clear conscience I apply myself to reply to your questions. Gladly undertake this small item for the good of the cause.'

The war brought about a heightened public appreciation of dental services that continued in peacetime. There were three main reasons. First, the large number of men rejected for military service because of dental disease had received publicity; the general public now took its oral health more seriously. Second, the services of the Dental Corps during the war had an indirect result in that unprecedented numbers of demobilized men from all branches applied for admission to the dental schools. Third, the professional organizations had managed to continue their programs of dental education of the public despite the war. Newspapers of the postwar period carried considerable information respecting dental health. Ernest Hemingway, who was then a reporter with the Toronto *Star*, wrote at least two effective articles on the subject before going to Paris and fame as a novelist.[7]

The dental schools quickly found themselves in an emergency. Student applicants were in large part men who had already lost several years through military service, and from patriotic motives alone great effort was expended to accommodate them. Yet even before the war had ended the schools were filled to capacity, largely with men already discharged from the forces. With demobilization, the flood of applicants overtaxed all available teaching facilities.

Some effort to establish an additional school in Quebec occurred during this period. An item in the minutes of the Quebec College of Dental Surgeons (1916) reads: 'the Bill for the incorporation of the Royal Dental School had been refused by the Legislature.' It has not, however, been possible to secure details related to this project.

During the war, the University of Alberta had considered organizing a course in dentistry, and in the fall of 1918 three students were accepted. The dental course was established under the Faculty of Medicine on a four-year basis, with the first two years at Alberta and, by agreement, the final two years at the Royal College of Dental Surgeons or McGill University. The following year, the number of applicants increased far beyond the capacity of the course, but it was not until 1923 that dentistry was recognized as a separate department at Alberta, with H.E. Bulyea as director.

In the fall of 1919, the Royal College of Dental Surgeons at Toronto had 375 qualified applicants for the first dental year. The school was equipped for maximum classes of eighty students. Over eighty per cent of the applicants were men who had served overseas in the forces, many for the full four years of war. The members of the Ontario Board had tried to prepare for this crisis, but with limited success. The previous year they had estimated, on the basis of annual increases in the number of applications, that the College would have to provide for 500 students in the session beginning in the fall of 1919 (actually there were 804). To meet this expected demand they had applied to the Ontario Government for a grant of $100,000 to build an addition to the school: the estimated cost of the addition was $150,000, and in its application the Ontario Board promised to raise the balance. In the spring of 1919 the government had refused to consider any such grant, on the grounds that grants had never been made to independent educational institutions and to accede to this application would set a dangerous precedent. The situation became critical as hundreds of applicants milled around the campus in the fall. Hurried meetings were held with government authorities. The cause of the returned soldier was dominant at the time, and the newspapers gave more support to the issue than dentistry had ever been able to enjoy before. A change of government facilitated action, and eventually the province did make the grant – not actually until February 1920, but in the meantime all returned soldiers were accepted.[8] Certain conditions were attached to the grant, the main one being that the school could not be sold without government permission. Later, the Ontario Government created the Ex-Service Men's Loan Fund, under the terms of which loans (repayable after graduation) were made to student veterans who were in need of financial assistance. This provision made completion of the course possible for a considerable number of future dentists.

A minority of Ontario dentists argued that in seeking this grant the profession was 'selling out' to the government. In today's society, when government support is sought so liberally, such protest may appear strange, but then a pride of ownership existed. The Toronto school had been operated for nearly fifty years by the profession and this was the first time that outside financial assistance had been sought, even though for several years leaders had been stating that the profession could not continue to support dental education alone. More general criticism on educational grounds was levelled at the school for accepting so many students beyond the capacity of its existing teaching facilities. Such criticism was just and many expediencies had to be utilized, but there were saving factors. Perhaps the chief was the student age level. These returned men were much older than normal undergraduates, considered their opportunity a privilege, and were keen to establish themselves in civilian life. However, expansion of this nature was avoided following the second world war.

The use of dental assistants (sergeants) during the war prompted renewed discussion respecting the use and training of dental auxiliaries. The first recorded action was a resolution adopted at the annual meeting of Quebec licentiates early in 1917, requesting the establishment of a training course for dental nurses, but no action followed. The following year, Dean Webster recommended to the Ontario Board that a course for dental assistants be established. This resulted in a one-year course for dental nurses at the Toronto school, which began in the fall of 1919 and continued until 1960.[9]

Special concessions were made for dental sergeants who wished to register in dental schools, but only a small percentage applied. However, the special wartime courses in which the sergeants had been trained did arouse interest. Representatives of an organization called the Ontario Prosthetic Dental Association made presentations to the Ontario Board in two successive years, requesting the establishment of a course for laboratory assistants. A committee of three representatives of this association and three Board members was set up to study the proposal, but there is no record of their report. This incident nevertheless represents the first effort to establish training of technicians for civilian purposes, and the beginning of a continuing problem.

As an outcome of proposals made by the research committee of the Canadian Dental Association at two successive meetings, the Canadian Dental Research Foundation was formed under federal charter in 1920. Financial support for dental research was negligible at the time. The foundation established a fund in honour and recognition of the service and sacrifice of Canadian dentists during the war. Under the energetic leadership of Wallace Seccombe, and of a board made up of dental representatives from all provinces, a financial campaign was organized: moneys collected were to be placed in a trust fund, with the net annual income to be paid to the foundation for use in the support of research activities. The profession responded well. Many dentists made sizeable contributions. In addition, dental students gave money; grants were made by dental organizations across the country; and surpluses from social and athletic activities were turned in. Contributions from outside the profession were disappointing, however. The general public were not as research-minded as today, and failed to appreciate the practical value to be obtained, not only for dentistry but for research in general. Consequently only a fraction of the proposed capital fund was attained, but this remains intact to the present time and is still in active use.

Perhaps the greatest value of the campaign did not lie in the amount of money collected, but in the awakening to the need for dental research which it stimulated. A number of highly qualified, research-minded graduates had developed. The schools possessed little financial means, if any, to assist these men in research activities, and practically no means of publishing their results existed. The foundation endeavoured to find solutions. It assisted the men in other ways as well, but its main activity was for some twenty years the publication and distribution of acceptable research bulletins, varying in size from pamphlets to a book of 125 pages.

The bulletins were quickly in demand from many parts of the world, and did much to establish dental research in Canada on a firm basis. In 1951, the foundation came under the administration of the Research Council of the Canadian Dental Association, from which it had originated, and continues to assist research actively.

The father of dental research in Canada was Harold Keith Box. He was a brilliant student, who graduated from the Royal College of Dental Surgeons in 1914 and immediately became a part-time member of the staff. He was appointed professor of dental pathology and periodontology in 1920, and a few years later became research professor of periodontology. While conducting a practice and serving on the staff, he engaged in intensive dental research requiring long hours of concentration. In 1920, he received from the University of Toronto the first degree of Doctor of Philosophy earned by a Canadian dentist. Of the bulletins published by the Canadian Dental Research Foundation, he was the author of twelve. His research spanned many areas, but he was principally acknowledged as an international leader in periodontology. During his career, he received many honours. By the time of his death in 1956, Toronto had

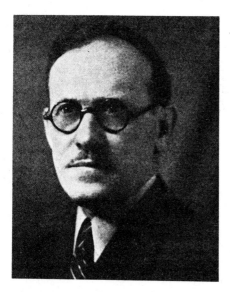

Harold Keith Box, DDS, PH D, father of
dental research in Canada

become well known as a centre of research in periodontics, and he left his work in the hands of a number of capable disciples.

Public dental health received some postwar assistance as one happy result of a great tragedy. On the morning of 6 December 1917, a ship loaded with explosives was rammed in the harbour of Halifax. The detonation dwarfed any previous disaster in Canada. Some 2,000 people were killed and 8,000 wounded. A large part of the city was devastated. All dental offices were more or less wrecked. None did more devoted relief work in hospitals, homes, or shelters than the dentists of the city. For a month, every dental office was practically closed and the entire time given to public needs. Immediate relief funds and supplies were made available from government and voluntary agencies. The Andrew Carnegie Commission offered to make good all damage to Dalhousie University. The neighbouring state of Massachusetts was very generous in making contributions. With moneys left over after relief needs had been taken care of, the Massachusetts-Halifax Health Commission was formed, for the purpose of conducting a public health campaign of education and pre-vention. Among its activities was the establishment of pre-school dental clinics, designed to render educational rather than reparative services. Arabelle Mackenzie, the first woman graduate in dentistry from Dalhousie University (1919), was placed in charge of the dental service with the title of pedodontist. Appointed in 1920, she was well qualified, having taken postgraduate training in the Forsythe Clinic at Boston. The project as a whole is notable in that the services concentrated upon the early ages, from prenatal to six years, with emphasis on nutrition. This was the first instance in Canada of what in later years came to be known as well-baby clinics.[10]

The 1918 annual meeting of the Canadian Dental Association was held in Chicago in co-operation with the National Dental Association (which became the American Dental Association in 1922). This is the only occasion when the Association has held its meeting outside Canada. The emphasis of the meeting was placed largely upon experiences of the profession during the war.

The years immediately preceding 1920 were dominated by war and postwar pressures and advances. The stature of the dental profession in-creased greatly. With more demand for dental services, new assessments were required. The population of Canada in 1919 was 8.75 million, and there were 2,590 dentists. The distribution of practitioners was not good.

In Ontario (with approximately one-third of the total population but almost half the dentists) there was one dentist for every 2,292 people. Quebec had only one dentist to 6,445 people, while in British Columbia the ratio was one to 3,438. Beyond this evident imbalance, there was the challenge of new techniques that had developed rapidly with the urgency of war. Developments in the surgical-prosthesis field were notable. The diagnostic potential of the x-ray became fully recognized, but the economics of the average dental office hardly permitted its use as yet. Improved means of anaesthesia became available. The need for reorientation of dental education was recognized, and this was to become the predominating issue during the following years.

12
Altered concepts of training
1920-1924

Ideas discussed and debated during the previous decade reached a cul-
mination in the early 1920s. Emphasis in education was placed upon the
fundamentals underlying the profession of dentistry rather than the
practical aspects of practice. More complicated techniques demanded
better understanding of fundamental principles; a public awakened to the
serious nature of dental disease placed greater responsibility upon the
dentist; and the position of the dentist as a professional man in society as
a whole called for an appropriate academic background. These were
matters of primary concern to the dental schools, and fortunately the
leaders in dental education acted with dispatch and in harmony.

They were strongly influenced by a survey of dental education in the
United States and Canada conducted by the Carnegie Foundation.[1] While
the report was not published until 1926, the survey was in progress over a
five-year period and many of the recommendations were well known in
advance and implemented before they were formally announced. The
report was prepared by William J. Gies, a former professor of biological
chemistry at Columbia University who had an interest in dental research,
and it had a continuing influence on the direction of dental education in
North America over a long period. From the beginning, dental education
in Canada and the United States has followed parallel lines. The dental
schools of both countries had co-operated through various representative
organizations: the Dental Faculties Association of Canada, organized in
1920, three years later became amalgamated with the National Association of Dental Faculties and the American Institute of Dental Teachers in
the new American Association of Dental Schools. (Reversing this trend,

the Association of Canadian Faculties of Dentistry was formed in 1967, a move reflecting the establishment of several new schools across the country and the enlargement of the older ones. However, the Canadian schools retained associate membership with the American Association of Dental Schools.) The close co-operation of the profession in the two countries from the beginning in the development of dentistry has been most beneficial to Canada, particularly in the area of dental education.

During the eighteenth and nineteenth centuries, when this continent was settled, it was natural that the immigrants brought with them the customs of their native lands. In general, these usages were modified gradually, but in the case of dentistry a definite breakthrough occurred. In Europe, with variations from country to country, dentistry developed under the aegis of the medical profession, and academic requirements for the practice of dentistry were set within the jurisdiction of the medical schools. In most of these lands a separation of the two professions eventually occurred, but this was an extremely slow process and today there are still a small number of countries in Europe where graduation from a medical school is a requirement for the practice of dentistry.

In North America, despite some long-lived misconceptions about the beginnings of dental education, there was no quarrel between the medical and dental professions. Though tales of disagreement recur disturbingly often, seldom will the statement be found that lectures on odontology were given as early as the 1820s by dentists who were members of the staff at the Medical and Chirurgical Faculty of Maryland. Horace B. Hayden was one of these and must be regarded as the pioneer of institutional dental teaching. At Maryland and similar medical schools, education in the necessary biological sciences was satisfactory but difficulty was experienced in providing for adequate technical training. Highly respected men, both medical and dental, endeavoured to secure adequate facilities for instructing the dental student in both the science of dentistry and its art of practice. The result was the founding of the first independent dental school in the world in 1840, the Baltimore College of Dental Surgery.[2] From this beginning, emerged the independent dental school which has prevailed on the North American continent and many other parts of the world.

Only on two occasions have serious differences arisen between Canada and the United States in dental education. Shortly after the turn of the century, an agreement was reached to increase the normal dental course from three to four years. The existing Canadian schools (Toronto and

Montreal) took this action. The American schools evidently had second thoughts and delayed for several years. The second matter had to do with the conferring of the doctorate degree. Under Canadian law, only universities were permitted to confer academic degrees; in the United States all chartered dental schools conferred the degree with or without university affiliation. The first of these differences meant that for some time a Canadian could save a year of study by taking the shorter course in the United States. The second difference prompted a scepticism and even hostility towards graduates of the American proprietary schools, which had no counterpart in Canada. Any effect these differences had on the development of dental education in the two countries was temporary. But, in those Canadian provinces wherein a dental school existed, drastic action was taken by licensing boards to prohibit practice by graduates of American schools, and this regrettable attitude, with its repercussions, proved to be a lasting one. The western provinces, having no dental schools, welcomed American graduates. In 1918, over eighty per cent of the dentists in British Columbia had graduated from dental schools in the United States.

By the 1920s, the future of dental education had become the prime subject of professional importance. All through the previous decade, the serious leaders of the profession had pointed out the need for improvement. Among them was Frank Woodbury, dean at Dalhousie University and recognized as the dean of Canadian dentists during this period. In 1920 he stated in an address, 'As the years pass and the importance of dentistry in the preservation of the health of the world is being recognized, and the larger responsibility is being placed upon the profession, the necessity of better preparation becomes more apparent. Better preliminary education must be required if we are to keep step and continue to merit the confidence of the public.'[3] The alterations taking place in the curricula of the dental schools made the financing of dental education more difficult, but an increasing number of leaders in the profession spoke frankly in support. In essence, these men said that if the dentist of the day and in the future was to hold his high place in the community and in public esteem, he must develop that mental attitude and breadth of vision which come from a training that is based on a solid foundation. Dean Webster, as editor of the *Dominion Dental Journal*, wrote many editorials on the need for change in dental education.

The ground had been well tilled. The profession was ready in support. An amazing number of major alterations in dental education took place in a short period. Most of them depended upon education preliminary to the dental course, and on a proper relationship with a university. The ingredients necessary for the professional education these leaders envisioned were to be found only within the disciplines of a university.

Canada had at the time four developed schools and one in embryo. By 1921, three were full faculties within their respective universities – Dalhousie, McGill, and Montreal. At Toronto, the discussions that had been held on numerous occasions over the years with the officials of the university respecting establishment of a dental faculty finally bore fruit. To understand that situation, it must be remembered that the Toronto school was owned by Ontario dentists and operated by them through the direction of the Board of Directors of the Royal College of Dental Surgeons of Ontario as trustees. There existed considerable pride of ownership. When a tentative agreement had been negotiated, the Ontario Board prepared and mailed out detailed explanatory circulars to the profession. In turn, what proved to be a small group of reactionary dentists also circularized their colleagues.[4] The whole matter was complicated by internal school matters, but when the Board submitted the proposed agreement to the membership, 858 out of 870 voting were in favour. Under the agreement, the building, fittings, and equipment valued at just under half a million dollars became the property of the university. This action by Ontario dentists portrays the profession at one of its finest hours. The Faculty of Dentistry of the University of Toronto was established in 1925, the fourth in Canada. The fifth, in Alberta, initially was formed as a division of the Faculty of Medicine in 1918. In 1923, it was operated as a department and eventually was recognized as a separate faculty of the University of Alberta in 1942.

One of the important alterations in the pattern of training was the instituting of a pre-professional course. The secondary school level was no longer adequate for admission to the study of dentistry; instead, students were required to take a set of subjects referred to as basic, cultural, and scientific. The Carnegie report later recommended that two years be required for this study and after considerable debate on various arrangements, the Canadian schools adopted what came to be known as the two-four plan – two years pre-dental and four years professional education. The change was gradual. In the fall of 1919, when the Toronto school was faced with an excessive number of applicants, it offered a one-year voluntary pre-professional course to those who could not be accepted in the professional course. Eighteen men accepted the opportunity. Two years later, the two-four plan was made compulsory at Toronto. At Dalhousie, the plan was adopted in 1922, and at McGill in 1925. The French-speaking school in Montreal faced a somewhat different situation. Most of its applicants came from the classical colleges of the province of Quebec. No question arose respecting the cultural content of the courses they had taken, but there existed considerable variation in the scientific content. Eventually the problem was overcome by requiring those applicants wanting in science to fulfill the requirements in a pre-professional course.

No longer could the mere mastery of technical skills be considered the only necessary qualification of the dentist. This change was of the utmost importance to the future of the profession. Great activity occurred within the dental faculties as they arranged their curricula to the new formula, with considerable variation in detail from school to school. A decade later, a curriculum survey committee was organized by the American Association of Dental Schools consisting of representatives of dental schools in the United States and Canada under the chairmanship of Dean Seccombe of Toronto. The report of this committee in 1935 set minimum requirements for content in the curriculum but in no way curbed the excellence of teaching in any particular branch of dentistry in any school. That report really completed, for the time being, the alteration of dental education begun in the early twenties.[5]

Among the many matters contained in the Carnegie Report, one other should be mentioned. From time to time some influential dentists have questioned the autonomous position of their profession in relationship to medicine. While there was never any question but that the majority of dentists stood for independence, there were strong arguments on both sides of the question. The report discussed this matter at considerable length and summarized its findings in the statement, 'That dentistry is an independent division of health service which is attaining the full equivalence of an oral specialty of medicine, and commends these views of the Foundation to the attention of the public and of the medical and dental professions.' This conclusion, heartily commended by dental bodies, brought to an end the recurring discussions on the subject until recent years, when it arose again in a different form.[6]

The effectiveness of changes made at this time in the pattern of dental education has been proven over the years. While many improvements in detail have since been made, the general outline has remained the same. The trend has been steadily to ever more education. A considerable number of students now enter the professional course with higher academic standing than the two year pre-professional course. More remarkable still has been the great increase in graduate education, which can be largely attributed to the foundation of dental education established in this period. The transition was not, however, as easy as it may appear. Objections were strong from those dentists who called themselves practical. It was said that dental schools would produce graduates who would know everything except how to practise. Strong leadership was fortunately at hand in the persons of the deans of the dental schools. Woodbury of Dalhousie, Thornton of McGill, Dubeau of Montreal, Webster and (after 1923) Seccombe of Toronto had ample reason to know that a profession is born Stoic and dies Epicurean.

In spite of the progress which had been made in the recognition of dentistry as a professional health service, threatening incidents still arose. One was related to taxation. In 1920 the federal government issued an order that dentists, as manufacturers, would have to pay the recently-introduced sales tax of two per cent. Protests were made by all dental organizations. To make matters worse, a subsequent order required dentists to obtain trading licences and cancelling machines for use in collecting the tax. While the amount of the tax was small, the principle involved was great: was dentistry a trade or truly a profession serving the public health? After considerable effort, the Canadian Dental Association succeeded in having the order abrogated. The decision reached at this time, after a strenuous battle by the profession, created a precedent, laying the foundation for future decisions in many areas, even in matters related to taxation.

The matter of legal aid for dentists facing actual or threatened malpractice actions became a subject of concern at this time. As early as 1917, the Ontario Dental Society had set up a committee to study the subject under the chairmanship of R.J. McLaughlin of Toronto. As a result of the committee's report, the Dentists' Legal Protective Association of Ontario was organized in 1923 and has acted in the interests of Ontario dentists ever since. On several occasions, efforts have been made to establish a similar organization on a national basis, but these endeavours have failed. Similar organizations have, however, been established in British Columbia and Alberta.

Focal infection – infection spreading throughout the circulation from circumscribed collections of bacteria – became a dominant theory for the cause of disease in the early 1920s. While several possible foci existed in the human body, the mouth came under most suspicion. The theory gained such support that the discovery of a devitalized tooth or a large restoration, particularly a gold crown, in a patient's mouth prompted many a medical practitioner to prescribe immediate extraction. The position of the dentist was very awkward. For a decade, focal infection appeared to be the most frequent diagnosis for almost any ailment. Many quips developed during this period. One was a new definition of a specialist, as a man who wants all your teeth pulled before he tries another guess.

The effect on dental practice was both good and bad. Large numbers of sound teeth were extracted needlessly and this was regrettable. On the other hand, the dentist was forced to improve his diagnostic ability. The x-ray became an essential aid. Improved root-canal therapy and new techniques for large restorations also resulted. Dentists were quick to respond to the focal infection challenge and its new requirements, but recognition that dentists were capable of making a proper scientific diagnosis of the mouth came about rather more slowly.[7] The relationship between tooth infection and general health had in fact been recognized for many years. The implementation in practice of the theory of focal infection as a cause of disease during this period often was based more on enthusiasm than reasoning. The pendulum swung altogether too often to the exclusion of other causes. Increased knowledge, better diagnostic methods, and improved techniques brought about a more scientific approach by the 1930s.

Measurement of the stature of a profession can be best estimated by the three recognized fundamentals; education, association, and journalism. Dental education in Canada was now on a solid foundation. Professional organizations had in many cases gone through adjustments, but by this time were well established, represented well their members at the local, provincial, and national levels, and were creditable scientific bodies. Journalistically, the profession was served by the English-language *Dominion Dental Journal* and *Oral Health*. The first issue of a journal in the French language had appeared in December 1915 under the editorship of Honoré Thibault. This publication first appeared as *La Société d'Odontologie* but the name was changed in the following May to *La Revue Dentaire Canadienne*. It continued to be published monthly until 1934, and eventually merged with the new *Journal of the Canadian Dental Association*. In 1926, the Ontario Dental Association began a monthly publication called *The Booster*. The name was altered to *The Journal of the Ontario Dental Association* in 1931 and it has been published continuously since.

An event of importance for the future was the appointment in 1924 of a director of dental services by the Ontario Government, the first government in Canada to do so. Ontario had already established a Department of Health in 1923 to replace the Provincial Board of Health – an action which had extended provincial activity in health matters and had prompted the Ontario Dental Association to intensify its long-term efforts to secure the appointment of a dental director. The first to hold the title was F.J. Conboy, an active, public-spirited man who held a great number of positions of trust within and without the profession during his lifetime. He served as president of both the Ontario and Canadian Dental Associations and was secretary of the provincial body for fifteen years. For twenty-nine years, he was a lecturer on the staff of the Toronto school. In public life he served in many capacities, including the mayoralty of Toronto for two terms. He died in 1949. As director of dental services, he ardently advanced the cause of dental health within his province. His appointment was the beginning of the establishment of dental divisions within departments of health, though it was to take twenty-five years before all Canadian governments had taken similar action.

The first report in the literature of what came to be called industrial dentistry appeared in 1924.[8] The Laurentide Health Service had been established at Grand'Mère, Quebec, in 1922, and was notable for emphasis on dental health. Its dental clinic was in charge of a dental hygienist trained at the Forsythe Dental Infirmary at Boston, the first member of this auxiliary vocation known to have been employed in Canada. The services performed at the clinic were described in the *Dominion Dental Journal* as 'an examination of the mouth to see the condition of the teeth and a thorough cleansing of the mouth and teeth and where pyorrhea has set in, treatment for pyorrhea is given. The condition of the mouth is charted and where there is work for the dental surgeon indicated, the man is urged to go at once to some dentist ...' Accurate records were kept and for the first two years a tremendous improvement in dental health among employees was recorded. A great deal of discussion occurred in future years as to the services properly rendered by industrial dental clinics.

The Harry R. Abbott Memorial Library was established in 1925, one of the first philanthropic actions taken by a dentist in the interests of his profession. Harry Abbott graduated from the Toronto school in 1901, received his dental degree from Trinity, and engaged in practice in London, Ontario. For 25 years he was a member of the Ontario Board, as well as occupying many other noteworthy professional positions. On his death in 1921, it was found that his will provided for the establishment and maintenance of a dental library, the trust fund to be administered by the Board of the Royal College of Dental Surgeons of Ontario. By agreement, this library is housed at the Faculty of Dentistry of the University of Toronto and remains a continuing memorial to a man who served his profession well.

Marked professional progress had been made in the stabilization of dental education under university control, but some less salutary professional matters still required regulation. Among these was advertising. From the beginning, flagrant and objectionable advertising had been a thorn in the flesh of ethical practitioners. In all provinces, blatant newspaper advertisements, large signs, showcases at entrances to dental offices, distribution of advertising cards, and other means had been utilized by a small minority to the detriment of the profession as a whole. Amendments to the provincial dental acts were sought and obtained, but no sooner was one loophole plugged than offences appeared in another form. The matter became political in some provinces. In Nova Scotia in 1919, one of these advertisers obtained an amendment permitting him (and others) to employ unregistered assistants in his dental parlour. The Quebec Board spent a considerable sum in legal fees to bring the objectionable activities of the Institut Dentaire Franco-American at Montreal under control. During the twenties the showcases at the entrances to dental offices along Yonge Street in Toronto came down through action by the Ontario Board. The battle was long and arduous. Through good legal advice it was eventually won, but spasmodic cases continued to arise for several years. The creation over a long period of controlling regulations for ethical conduct of practice contributed, second only to dental education, to the advancement of the profession.

By 1925, Canada had approximately 3,600 dentists to serve 9.5 million people. Ontario had 51 per cent of the dentists to serve 40 per cent of the population, while British Columbia had 5.5 per cent to serve 5 per cent of the population. The number of dentists had increased considerably as a result of the large classes accepted in the schools following the first world war. The overall ratio of dentists to population was higher than it would be for many years to come. During the depression the student level in the schools was to reach a low ebb while the population continued to increase; and no new training facilities for dentists were to be established in Canada until another war had passed.

Thomas Cowling was a writer far above average in ability. After graduating in dentistry, he gained his master's degree in Arts and later his doctorate in paedagogy, which was certainly unusual for a dentist of the time. He was a member of the staff of the Toronto school for thirty-seven years, serving as assistant dean for eight years previous to his death in 1950. For fourteen years, he was editor of *Oral Health*. In 1924, Cowling published a detailed review of the existing status of dentistry. His report was optimistic: 'We recall that only a few years ago, we were clamoring for recognition; today more attention is being given to dentistry than to any other branch of the healing art. Quite truthfully, it may be said that the past few years have been years of great achievement and noted also for the hopefulness of outlook.'[9] This statement represents the spirit and attitude of the time.

13

Public health

1925-1929

The Canadian Dental Hygiene Council was incorporated by federal charter in 1924. Its sixteen stated objectives were all-embracing, but in reality the first indicated the purpose: 'To undertake such measures as may be necessary to prevent, reduce or assist in the control of dental disease, thus establishing a higher standard of public health.' The original sponsors envisioned an organization broad in scope with public participation, thus widening the base of an activity which up to this time had been sponsored by the profession with very little outside assistance, government or otherwise. The interest and participation of outstanding lay citizens contributed greatly to the success of the council. For over twenty years, it functioned successfully and must be given credit for establishing public health dentistry on a firm basis in Canada.[1]

In a country as large as Canada, there is much room for variation from province to province. The first recorded efforts to render dental services to the public at large, other than through private practice, had occurred before the turn of the century in Nova Scotia (the Halifax Visiting Dispensary) and Ontario (Christ's Mission Dental Hospital). As related earlier, the charitable work of J.G. Adams in Toronto ended in a tax dispute, but the Halifax Visiting Dispensary operated until the 1920s, when it was replaced by school dental clinics. These endeavours had a lasting influence far beyond the actual treatment they rendered. They aroused the interest both of the public and of the profession. Dentists began to realize that treatment alone was not the complete answer to the problems of dental health: an intensive program directed towards the education of the public was also essential. As a consequence, the dental organizations in these two provinces established committees during the early 1900s to educate the public. This action was followed gradually in other provinces. Through the years, the title given these committees is indicative of progressive thinking. Initially known as 'education' committees, they became 'oral hygiene' committees during the second decade and then 'dental public health' committees during the latter twenties. They were active in utilizing all possible media towards the education of the public, and at the same time in arousing the profession to the need. To a considerable degree the increasing stature of dentistry is attributable to their enthusiastic efforts.

A notable event occurred in Quebec during the mid-twenties when, under the leadership of Joseph Nolin, a commission on dental hygiene was set up with financial support from the provincial government. Nolin was a well-respected dentist, vice-dean of dentistry at l'Université de Montréal, a past president of the Canadian Dental Association, and above all a most capable man. The commission made a thorough study of activities by the profession in public education, and visited the main centres in the United States and Canada to gain information. Its report, when read today, has a modern ring, setting forth the mistakes of the past and pointing out directions for future activities.[2] Nolin pointed out that the informative literature then being distributed was intelligible to dentists but not adapted to the public for whom it was intended; that much of the information distributed was contradictory; that in all the visits made by the commission little proof was found for the statements being made; that the base of operation had to be broadened by gaining the interest of public health officials, the medical profession, and leading public-minded citizens; and that the responsibility for the movement toward preventive dentistry was the dental profession's. He pointed out in a frank manner that the average dentist took little personal interest in public education and was willing to relegate the responsibility to a few individuals while he remained a critical spectator.

A turning point in the movement for public health dentistry had been reached. Assessments were also taking place in the other provinces, particularly in Ontario. The truth of the statements made by Nolin were attested by future programs of public education. It was during this reassessment period that the Canadian Dental Hygiene Council came into being.

It was in one sense an offshoot of the Canadian Oral Prophylactic Association which since 1906 had raised money, through the sale of recommended dentifrices and tooth brushes, to finance public education and dental research. In 1920, Harry S. Thomson of New Brunswick had been appointed director of that association. Thomson was a graduate of Tufts Dental College in 1906, and a former president of the New Brunswick Dental Society. He was a most capable organizer and inspirational speaker. But in the association he quickly found himself facing the old dilemma of an organization engaged in commercial activities and professional pursuits at the same time. In solution of the problem, and to enlarge dental public health activity, Thomson conceived the idea of a separate Canadian Dental Hygiene Council, and secured the interest of the profession and a number of prominent laymen. He was appointed field secretary of the newly-formed council. For twenty-four years, he directed a campaign of education in dental public health which bore abundant fruit both for the public and the profession. When the main objectives had been accomplished, he retired.

For several years, the Canadian Oral Prophylactic Association lent their director to the council, paying his salary. Initial financial support was difficult, but came from many sources including governments, the Red Cross, dental organizations, and the Canadian Life Insurance Officers Association. Improved educational information was produced and distributed through all possible media. The most important activity was the

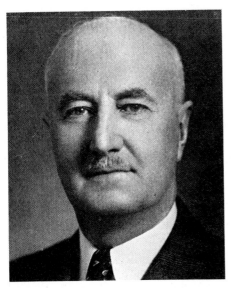

Harry Scott Thomson, DMD, Field
Secretary, Canadian Dental Hygiene Council

Mouth Health Campaigns in the provinces. The first of these took place in Saskatchewan in 1928. The province was divided into sections, with a committee in each section made up of lay representatives together with one or two local dentists. The field secretary visited each section before the campaign to help with plans. Through its Departments of Health and Education, the Saskatchewan Government participated, and so did the Canadian Red Cross and other lay organizations. A travelling dental clinic was used to reach outlying areas. In the course of each campaign, the mouths of the area's school children were examined by dentists, and lay organizations of all kinds were addressed. It was said that the entire province thus took a course in preventive dentistry. This overall approach was new, received co-operative support, and proved to be the most successful effort in dental public health up to that time. In following years, similar campaigns, with some variations, were conducted in the other provinces.

In the beginning there were no means to build a continuing program once a campaign was over. Recognizing this weakness, the council set as one of its earliest objectives the establishment of a division of dental health in each government health department, with a properly qualified director in charge, as already existed in Ontario. When the council surrendered its charter in 1948, it could announce with understandable pride that this main objective had been achieved. Here was an organization formed to meet a definite public need, which accomplished its objective and then of its own accord ceased to exist. Governments had assumed the responsibility, and professional organizations had strengthened their activities in dental public health to a point where the cause could be carried forward without it.

Within the profession, the council also gave fine leadership. Practically all dental organizations formed active committees on dental public health. Indeed, outside of the scientific programs, dental public health became the dominant activity of many professional organizations. Two provinces formed special organizations to carry on the work. In Manitoba, the Canadian Foundation for Preventive Dentistry was formed in 1929 with the full support of the Manitoba Dental Association, and carried on an active program for several years. For some reason, this foundation was organized under a federal charter, but confined its activities to Manitoba. In Quebec, after several arrangements, the Ligue d'Hygiène Dentaire de la Province de Québec, Inc, was incorporated and continues to carry out an extensive program.

When John G. Adams wrote his letter to the Ontario Board of Health in 1896, he was initiating a policy of dental care for children which has been adhered to, with variations, ever since. Before that he had operated his dental hospital for twenty-three years, done considerable travelling to other municipalities, and investigated dental health conditions in other countries. The need for action was compelling. The record, fortunately extant, suggests that while Adams was staunchly supported by the Toronto Dental Society, it was the ardent demand for action by the Toronto Trades and Labour Council that influenced the Provincial Board of Health to carry out a detailed study and recommend the periodic inspection of school children's teeth. Of course, action on the recommendation was slow, but by the end of the 1920s, most larger urban municipalities across Canada had some form of dental inspection for children, with arrangements for dental care for those whose parents could not pay.

This whole movement was part of a slowly growing recognition of government responsibility for public health. Today's great interest in the field, including the jurisdictional arguments between Ottawa and the provinces, is a comparatively recent development. The British North America Act of 1867, often referred to as Canada's constitution, made extremely little reference to health, except to state that the federal government would maintain marine hospitals and that provincial governments were responsible for the establishment, maintenance, and management of hospitals, asylums, charities, and eleemosynary institutions, other than marine. The first department of health in Canada was established by New Brunswick in 1918, an example followed gradually by the federal government and other provinces.[3] Previously, provincial boards of health had existed, more or less indirectly related to the legislatures. These boards were rather circumscribed in their duties and limited respecting any financial assistance. It is perhaps fair to state that up to the establishment of departments of health, advances made in health care were attained by the professions with only meagre assistance from government. Indeed representatives of the dental profession had difficulty even in approaching government. In one province, the Department of Agriculture, strange to say, proved to be the most helpful government agency for several years. Because school children were the chief target of the programs of preventive dentistry, the Department of Education was the one most often approached, and generally proved co-operative. With the establishment of departments of health, the line of approach became clearer. But even so, government activities were not enough: the profession has remained active in the field, creating and distributing information about the importance of prevention and dental public health.

Since the early 1900s, the watchword of Canadian dentistry has been prevention. It is true that many preventive theories for dental diseases have arisen and waned. The profession has always endeavoured to secure adequate proof before advocacy. With the advancement of dental research, the position in this respect has become more secure than was the case in earlier days.

In 1927, seven students graduated in dentistry after taking the first complete course offered at the University of Alberta. The course had been started in 1918 as part of the Faculty of Medicine. The initial instructor was H.E. Bulyea, who had been born in New Brunswick, graduated from Harvard Dental School in 1897, and after practising a few years in his home province, moved to western Canada where he became greatly respected, both as a man and a dentist. As this was written he was still living – despite the fact that as early as 1903 he was already president of the New Brunswick Dental Society, and even before that had been chosen to present clinics to meetings of that society.[4] He piloted the Alberta school from birth until its establishment as a faculty in 1942, when he retired. Many honours have been bestowed upon him, including the degree of Doctor of Laws by the University of Manitoba. A more than

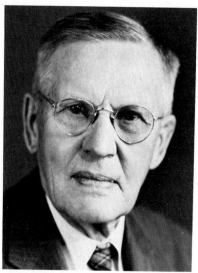

H.E. Bulyea, DDS, LLD, Director of the
Dental Department, University of
Alberta, 1918–42

ordinary point is the great respect in which his former students hold this grand old man of Canadian dentistry.

The establishment and sustaining of a national organization in a federated country like Canada is difficult, even without the geographical separation and diverse interests of a people spanning four thousand miles from coast to coast. In its development, the Canadian Dental Association by this time had tried several arrangements to ensure satisfactory representation and financing, none of which had proved very successful. The progress of the Association depended largely upon the faithful few who gave generously of both time and money. Under such conditions, the many important accomplishments of the Association appear amazing. Few questioned the need for a strong national organization, but the means to provide the necessary financial support were a subject of endless debate. In 1926, John Clay of Calgary, a highly respected dentist, was elected president and undertook a reorganization of the Association on a more equitable basis. It would be difficult to find a more active period in the history of the presidency than his two years. Several of the provincial bodies in this period felt self-sufficient, and Clay had difficulty securing the participation of a representative body in every province. He did achieve this, however. Financial support on a per capita basis also was attained, though at this stage it was minimal, and indeed insufficient. A new constitution was drafted, and adopted in 1928 – another step forward. However, the Association waited another decade before a new effort built upon Clay's work established a truly sound basis of operation. The day of commercial air travel had not arrived, and the time and expense involved in transportation was still a great handicap. Ways had to be be found to take the Association to the membership, rather than expecting the members to come to it.

By the 1920s, the older settled parts of Canada were well served by health personnel. But there were other enormous, sparsely settled areas with little or no medical or dental services at all. Co-operative endeavours by the profession with the departments of health and lay organizations, chiefly the Canadian Red Cross, sought to overcome this want. Railroad coaches to serve small municipalities along the right of way, and motor coaches for other areas, were equipped as travelling dental offices. In the most remote areas, dentists and equipment were carried by any means available.

Arrangements varied from province to province to meet existing conditions. The first rural treatment program apparently was organized in

Nova Scotia. Red Cross caravans – consisting of equipped ambulances staffed by a dentist, a nasopharyngeal specialist, a public health physician, and a public health nurse – toured remote areas of the province during the summer months for several years, beginning in 1919. Two years later Saskatchewan, through the Junior Red Cross, organized dental coaches for the same end. Other provinces followed. In Alberta, Government Travelling Clinics were organized in 1924 and operated until the war years, when the shortage of personnel forced them to stop. One who took part in this service wrote:[5]

The Travelling Clinic was organized in the late twenties to give medical and dental treatment to the children of the rural areas of the province. At that time practically all the outlying areas were without medical and dental treatment and the need was great.

The staff of the clinic consisted of one surgeon and one anaesthetist, two dentists, five nurses and a truck driver. Transportation was by automobile and truck, and in some instances when neither automobile nor truck were available the staff was forced to use animals to transport their equipment. Difficulties of travelling were legend with the clinic, however, regardless of travelling inhibitions the clinic managed to be considerably prompt in carrying out its schedule. In some instances the staff was forced to play the part of the woodsman and road builder. This held true especially in wet weather when travelling over the infamous dirt roads of the rural provincial areas. To compensate for the bad surfaces the members laid willow and small poplar trees on the road to get through. In most instances there was an itinerary of the areas the clinic was to visit. A district nurse was assigned to each area and she would arrange a schedule of patients for her particular area. This same nurse made the necessary arrangements for working accommodations, which were usually a school or church. Tents were on the average the living quarters for the staff.

The most frequent patients were farmers' children, however, in the sparsely populated North, the clinic often came in contact with trappers and Indians.

The tentative schedule for the group was to examine Thursday, operate Friday and move Saturday. The restorative dental program lasted four days, since there was no laboratory work. The dental equipment consisted of two portable chairs, portable dental cabinets, instruments and two foot engines.

The restorative progress consisted of amalgams and silicates. Most of the extractions were done under a general anaesthesia and usually in association with a tonsillectomy.

Often, there would be as many as fifty general anaesthetics in a single operating day, using ethyl chloride and ether. As you can well imagine, treatment was under the most primitive conditions, but there was never the first casualty.

During the 1920s, considerable enthusiasm developed for dental research, but it was soon realized that enthusiasm alone would accomplish little. The real need was twofold – more financial support and more qualified personnel. In 1926, the Canadian Dental Research Foundation reported that it had granted small sums to the Toronto and Halifax schools; the other schools had intimated they were not yet ready to undertake research. The work at Dalhousie was of a minor nature but, through much effort and sacrifice, more satisfactory progress was taking place at Toronto under the leadership of Harold K. Box. His PHD in pathology demonstrated the need for graduate study and higher degrees in dentistry. In 1927 the University of Toronto established the degrees of Bachelor of Science in Dentistry, BSC (DENT), and Master of Science in Dentistry, MSC(DENT). While these graduate programs did not solve all difficulties, they did establish a sound academic foundation for the training of researchers and the carrying out of their endeavours.[6]

One other man among the early researchers at Toronto deserves mention. W.E. Cummer did monumental work in dental prosthetics, introducing engineering principles to establish order out of chaos. Cummer was born in Hamilton, Ontario, and registered in dentistry at Toronto. He was an excellent student and almost immediately after graduation in 1902 became a member of the staff. He was appointed professor of prosthetics in 1907, a position he held for twenty-four years. In 1931, he was appointed dean of the School of Dentistry at the University of Detroit. Two years later, while at the very height of his dental career, he resigned the deanship and was admitted to the Basilian novitiate, and was ordained as a priest in 1938. He had a life-long interest in music. In dentistry, music, or religion, he was a perfectionist. Professionally he was greatly in demand as a clinician and had an international reputation. Few dentists have exceeded his contribution to dental literature.

In 1928, Dentistes de Langue Française de l'Amérique du Nord was organized, with S. Gaudreau as president, to bring together French-speaking dentists in Canada and the United States. It began with great enthusiasm, but owing to development of parallel organizations during these years, much of its support was dissipated and it disappeared after holding seven congresses, the last of them at Quebec City in 1941.[7]

The first recorded survey of Canadian dentists was made by the Royal College of Dental Surgeons of Ontario during 1929.[8] Presumably the results may be taken to reflect more or less the situation in the other provinces as well. Approximately one-quarter of Ontario dentists returned completed questionnaires consisting of over fifty questions. The answers to a few of these questions indicate the nature of dental practice at that time. Less than half the dentists reporting employed a lady assistant or nurse. The average gross income reported was $5,864.75, the average net income being $3,576.51. It is interesting to note that only 25 per cent of patients paid regular fees, and 3.5 per cent paid no fee at all. Two-thirds of the dentists inserted gold foil fillings. Practically all encouraged parents to bring their children to the dental office. Just under 40 per cent made use of commercial dental laboratories. Approximately one-third of practice time was occupied with prosthetic dentistry, and the average fee for full vulcanite dentures was $53.08. Some 60 per cent of the dentists made use of a recall system for patients. Very few dentists used an operating stool. No mention of x-ray is contained in this detailed survey, and other sources confirm that comparatively few dental offices had x-ray equipment at the time.

A persistent subject in dental records over many years was reciprocity of licence. Pro-British sentiment was strong in Canada, and efforts were made to obtain some form of mutual recognition of graduates of both countries. This movement was initiated by the Royal College of Dental Surgeons of Ontario in the 1880s and continued to be discussed by correspondence. Other provinces became interested, and in 1912 the Canadian Dental Association appointed a committee to pursue the matter. In May 1930, Matthew A. Garvin, a past president of the Canadian Dental Association, represented the profession at a conference in London, England, called by the British Dental Association and attended by several representatives from the Dominions and Colonies.[9] No tangible result for Canadian dentistry resulted, and indeed the difficulties involved respecting reciprocity appear to have been great. The form and content of dental training, as developed in North America, differed considerably from that in Great Britain. In addition, the British seemed to have difficulty understanding licensing powers by provinces in a federated country. In Canada, a form of reciprocity had been achieved between provinces through the Dominion Dental Council, but unfortunately two provinces did not recognize the certificate of the Council and this fact proved another stumbling block. From time to time discussions have continued, but up to the time this was written no form of reciprocity with British dental authorities had been achieved. History provides no alternatives, but the question arises as to the effect on the development of Canadian dentistry had reciprocity been won during these long negotiations.

The latter 1920s were prosperous years. The industrial boom of the mid-twenties gave rise to a psychosis of speculation and an over-extension of credit which led to inflated prices. Enthusiasts thought the economy had transcended the process of boom and slump. Dentistry had progressed along with the general economy, reaching a pinnacle of service to the population by the end of the decade. The economic disaster ahead was not suspected. But dentists would learn in the thirties that, unlike some other needs, dental care can be neglected when money is short. The profession was about to face a most difficult period.

14
Depression years
1930-1934

The Great Depression came with unprecedented abruptness and speedily worsened. The unsophisticated citizen could not understand why transactions on distant stock exchanges should bring calamity to him, and he had a deep suspicion that the experts didn't know either. The causes of the economic crisis are still being debated. The 1920s had been a decade of great expansion, accompanied by increased production and rising prices. Stocks rose by 25 per cent in 1928 and 35 per cent during the early months of 1929. Great numbers of people bought stocks on very low margin, seeing no reason why they should not participate in the enormous profits they visualized. Investments became dangerously speculative, with shares in industry being priced far beyond their value. Commodities sold easily at inflated prices. The crisis came on 24 October 1929, 'Black Thursday,' when the pendulum swung far in the opposite direction, bringing financial ruin to a great many persons, drastic cut-backs in industry, accompanying unemployment, and a fall in commodity prices below the cost of production. The situation worsened during the early thirties, with ever more people desperately attempting to find a means of livelihood. A full decade was to pass before Canada recovered from this economic catastrophe, world-wide in its scope and unequalled in history in its impact. Governments undertook solutions, radical and on a scale undreamed of previously. All kinds of ideas were advanced, both wise and unwise, and solutions were recommended by many a newly-formed organization. The proposals varied from complete socialism to stringent free enterprise.

Like everyone else, members of the health professions were severely affected. Many, deeply in debt and serving patients who themselves had no money, were ruined financially. The payment of an account in actual money became a significant event. Barter was the system of the day, and patients brought whatever they could spare in exchange for services. Yet few patients asked for or accepted charity. The great majority either found some method of recompense for services rendered, or paid their debt at a later date, sometimes years afterward. In dental practice, the most regrettable result was neglect – patients put off treatment rather than build up a debt which could not be paid.

As in other countries, Canadian governments, both federal and provincial, were faced with the problem of providing for the unemployed. Health services constituted a sizeable part of this responsibility, and brought government into an area it had not previously entered. Health service schemes varied somewhat from province to province, but in general all experienced difficulties in establishing a satisfactory means of administration both for patients and for practitioners. In the midst of these difficulties, and with costs of administration rapidly rising, the medical profession in Ontario approached the government and offered to take over the administration of medical services at a stated per capita rate of payment. This proposal was accepted and proved more satisfactory to all concerned. This was the initiation of a system which spread to several other provinces as a basis for managing future health service plans. During the early stage the dental profession co-operated in this arrangement, but later it withdrew, deciding that the two health services did not mix well administratively. Dental services during the depression were administered in Ontario by a government advisory committee made up of dentists. Various other systems operated in the other provinces. In the larger urban centres, dental societies were instrumental in setting up free clinics, in which large numbers of their members gave voluntary service.

By 1931, there were dentists on relief. Practice in rural areas was carried on largely by barter of commodities for services: many a dentist had the backyard of his home piled high with wood for use in his coal-burning furnace and his cellar filled with edibles accepted as payment. The worst conditions existed in industrial areas, where the large number of unemployed had nothing to offer. The depth of the depression was reached in 1933. After that conditions improved, but very gradually. These trying conditions were met with a sense of humour, as in the case of the farmer patient who assured his dentist that he would be able to pay in cash when he sold his pigs: when the dentist observed how nice it was to have pigs ready for market, the farmer replied that the old sow wasn't pregnant yet.

The area most afflicted was in the Prairie provinces, centred in Saskatchewan, where the depression coincided with the great drought. During five or six years of little rain, hot dry winds, and no crops, the people lived on hope. 'Prosperity is just around the corner' was the famous saying. Dentists, like everyone else, suffered great hardships. One in Saskatchewan has left a summary of his experiences. He was the only dentist within a radius of forty miles and, he said, he did no more than any other dentist would have done. Proud mothers were compelled to bring their crying children for help and, with tears in their eyes, explain that they had no money; they always asked for a bill, for they did not want charity. This is what he received in barter: 'a thoroughbred Angus bull, 200 live hens and many dead ones, 50 turkeys, 20 ducks and geese, 100 lbs of butter, fresh pork and sausage, sauerkraut, a cellar always full of vegetables, a cook stove, a heater stove, a blacksmithing outfit, a lot of groceries, a mower, a wagon, an Essex coupe with rumble seat, a garage, 5 sets of team harness, 3 horse collars, 4 bridles, a saddle, 30 head of cattle, 13 horses, 6 live pigs and one dead one, 8 tons of hay, etc.' As he explains, the dentist himself had to become a barter man, trading the variegated goods he received to meet his necessities.[1] It is little wonder that in this area the era is still referred to as the Dirty Thirties.

To a greater or lesser degree, the whole country was affected. The Langstroth family at Saint John, New Brunswick, had been long established in dental practice – S.F. Langstroth from 1896 to 1906 and his son, L.A. Langstroth, from 1900 to 1930. Both were graduates of the Philadelphia Dental College. One of the third generation, R.S. Langstroth, having graduated from Toronto, joined his father in 1929. There was little dentistry to be practised. His father was well known for his hobby of collecting such things as coins, stamps, and documents, and the dental office quickly became an exchange place. People often were lined up on the sidewalk with valued possessions brought for sale. Practice of dentistry occurred chiefly in the evenings, because patients with jobs would not even think of requesting time off for a daytime appointment.[2]

These examples may have been more extreme than the average but all dentists were drastically affected. The degree of hardship depended upon location and type of practice. In general, the income of the specialist was more seriously reduced than that of the general practitioner.

Governments were hard pressed in all directions. Proposals for changing the administration of health services, and for adopting state health services or health insurance, were made by many lay organizations. Under the desperate economic conditions, the health professions agreed to greatly reduce fee schedules under government-sponsored schemes. Advertisers, attempting to take advantage of the public, became active again with a new wrinkle – mail-order dentistry. Some legislative changes occurred, the most important of them from the standpoint of dentistry in Alberta. There, in 1933, the Public Health Act was amended, without consultation with the dental profession, to enable a registered dentist to be associated with a dental mechanic by means of a contract approved by the Provincial Board of Health. The contract had to include a description of the separate duties to be performed by each of the associates. The arrangement lent itself to abuses and was contrary to the accepted principle of control of the service by qualified practitioners. This action alarmed the dental profession in all provinces and constituted the beginning of a real problem of finding a proper relationship between dentist and dental technician.

Organizations representing the profession made various arrangements with government to provide dental services, in which the majority of dentists co-operated. But these agreements were not always to the liking of all the dentists concerned. Rugged individuals reacted vigorously to some measures. At one stage, the Alberta Dental Association agreed with the provincial government to supply dentures at a very low set fee in order to meet public needs, and sent out a circular letter to this effect to its members. One of them, William J. Greene of Peace River, took exception to being told what fee he would charge, and took a quarter page in the *Northern Gazette* to state his position in no uncertain terms. The association attempted to bring him in line but not very successfully.

Greene had an exceptional career. The main source of information about him is an abundance of newspaper clippings. He was born in San Francisco in 1872, apparently into a family of considerable means. He had an inventive turn of mind, and early in life turned his efforts towards inventing a machine which would fly. At the same time he attended the University of California, graduating in 1907 in both dentistry and medicine. For a time he practised dentistry in New York City, but spent most of his time inventing and experimenting with flying machines. He established himself as one of the three great rivals in the aviation industry, along with the Wright Brothers and Glenn Curtis, and was one of the first eight men to fly. He established several 'firsts.' Without having seen anyone fly, he built a plane and flew it for five hundred feet, a record at the time. In

1908 he became the first pilot to carry two passengers in a heavier-than-air machine, and received an outstanding award for this accomplishment. He established the first factory for the commercial production of airplanes at Rochester, NY, but then in a lawsuit lost his own money and that of friends who had backed him. Discouraged, he decided to get away as far as possible. In 1912 he arrived in the Peace River area and took up practice. After the declaration of war in 1914, he offered his services for training flyers and served briefly at Deseronto and Camp Borden airfields, but at this point in the fighting the Canadian Government was not greatly interested in air activities or else did not recognize the value of the man. In any event, he was discharged on account of age. Immediately, he offered his services to Washington and was made receiving and testing officer at the famous Kelly Field. Following the war, Greene returned to Peace River, turned his inventive mind to motor boats, and became a leader in conservation efforts. He continued to practise dentistry until his death in 1952. His widow erected a monument high above the town near the monument of the local folk hero, 'Twelve Foot Davis.'

As the depression continued, there was increased public criticism of the financial and economic institutions of the country. In 1933, the Canadian Dental Association submitted a resolution which had been approved by the provincial dental bodies to the prime minister. After stating that the current crisis afforded a special occasion for examining existing economic structures; that the laws regulating the promotion and administration of companies were in need of correction; and that the Canadian Dental Association was desirous of helping and supporting the country's statesmen, the resolution stated: [3]

because we do not wish to see a regime, sound in its source and principles, tend to eventually vanish away in almost general disapprobation, the Canadian Dental Association does herewith suggest to the Government of Canada the desirability of creating a NATIONAL COMMISSION composed of economists, jurists and professional men, not connected with politics or any financial group, for the purpose of investigating our present economic structure, with the end in view of recommending to Parliament the necessary changes for the removal of whatever is vitiated.

It will be observed that this resolution makes no mention of health services. Throughout the depression period, the emphasis was on economics and every organization in the country was under pressure to do something.

Specifically what was to be done was seldom definitely stated. Other organizations sent resolutions advising government action, but the fact remains that a commission such as was recommended in this resolution was set up and will be dealt with later.

Needless to say, there was little material progress during the early depression years, but professional advancement continued. Attendance at conventions was surprisingly good, and activities in the local societies increased considerably as dentists attempted to meet the need for service. Public health dentistry was not curtailed. When the Ontario Government, for economic reasons, dismissed its director of dental services, W.G. Thompson of Hamilton, a prominent dentist and former president of the Ontario Dental Association, took up the position on a voluntary basis and served four years until the government found it possible to make another appointment. Many dentists across the country assumed responsibilities without recompense, and often outside the scope of their profession, to meet needs of their communities. Considerable study was given to ways and means of providing services at fees patients could pay without reducing the quality of the service. Yet scientific advancement was not impaired, as programs at conventions illustrate. The number of students attending dental schools was, however, greatly reduced.

Within the profession it was a time of reassessment. Many dentists had time on their hands. In financial desperation, a few resorted to questionable methods of practice. In his 1930 presidential address to the Ontario Dental Association, A.W. Ellis said: 'There is an element of commercialism which creeps into our profession here and there, like a thief in the night. It robs the profession of that high ideal for which we exist and creates in the public mind a wrong and unpleasant attitude toward us, as members.' The first duty of a dentist, he continued, was to render service to the public to the best of his ability, and the great majority of the dental profession did place service first and fees second.[4] Ample evidence existed in support of his latter statement. Undoubtedly, dentists rendered more services, without consideration of payment, during this period than in any other. With time and good leadership available, more dentists also gave freely of their abilities in the field of dental public health, which became an asset in future years.

In the midst of these strained economic conditions, there occurred the most successful dental gathering in Canada up to the time. In 1932, a joint convention of the British Dental Association, Canadian Dental Association, and Ontario Dental Association was held at Toronto. Preparations had been made long in advance. Indications were few that the depression reduced attendance, for the registration was beyond anticipation. Some 145 notable representatives of the profession from Britain, the United States, and Canada presented papers and clinics – the greatest effort by dentistry to date at a convention in this country. During the meeting, the University of Toronto conferred the honorary degree of Doctor of Laws upon three prominent participants: George Northcroft of London, England, C.N. Johnson of Chicago, and Albert E. Webster of Toronto. An enlarged issue of the *British Dental Journal* was entirely devoted to reporting the meeting, and the editorial comment set forth with accuracy the attainments of Canadian dentistry at that time.[5]

The scientific basis of dental surgery and its practical application necessarily occupied an important place in the five days' deliberations and demonstrations, but it will be generally agreed that methods of prevention, and their predominating importance, were the outstanding feature of the meeting. Probably in no part of the world ... has dental hygiene been given a more prominent place by public authorities than in Canada, and it was not surprising to find that the officers of state who had honoured the gathering by participating in the programme, were insistent upon the desirability of including it in all official measures for public health.

In the lay press, the terms state medicine (or state dentistry) and health insurance appeared interchangeably during these years, with little interpretation of what was meant by either term, except that the government would pay. Understandably under such strained circumstances, some dentists were ready to support social change in the hope of improved conditions. Papers and editorials on the subject appeared in the dental journals. The following extracts from editorials in two such journals represent the diversity of opinion which existed.[6]

There are some dentists who feel that changes which in their opinion, must be made in the social order will lead to the introduction of a form of state dentistry. They apparently see the day when all dentists will be in the employ of the Government and all patients will attend clinics. No such thing will happen. There is no need for it. It could not be maintained except by direct provincial taxation and no government would think of introducing such a system.

And from another journal:

Believe it or not, like it or not, there is going to be some form of health insurance or health service under state control in every country of the world. Most countries even now have [some form of] state control of health. Dentistry has made out such a good case for the value of its services that the public, whether they pay for it or not, are going to demand it.

The first issue of the *Journal of the Canadian Dental Association* appeared for January 1935, with M.H. Garvin of Winnipeg as editor-in-chief and Philippe Hamel of Quebec as editor of the French section. S.A. Moore of London was business manager. The establishment of a national dental journal had been a subject of long negotiations. A committee for the purpose was set up during the 1920s but for several years reported only faltering progress. At the time there existed enough journals to serve the profession – The *Dominion Dental Journal, Oral Health, La Revue Dentaire Canadienne* and the *Journal of the Ontario Dental Association* – although only the last was actually published by and under the control of the profession. Much discussion took place, aimed at amalgamating all the journals into one national publication. This objective failed, and probably it was in the best interests of the profession that it did so for the expression of more than one viewpoint was a necessity. *La Revue Dentaire Canadienne* acquiesced in the proposal for a national journal, provided space was allotted in the publication for articles in French. Albert E. Webster had been editor of the *Dominion Dental Journal* for thirty-four years and took a good deal of pride in the publication, but after some hesitation he too decided it was best for the profession to possess its own journal. As a result of these decisions, the *Journal of the Canadian Dental Association* was inaugurated with the financial backing of the Association. Webster was appointed editor emeritus and after a brief period, Alcide Thibaudeau replaced Philippe Hamel as editor of the French section. With the new publication, the profession brought dental journalism under its control.[7]

Three men made a fine contribution to the advancement of the profession by their persistent efforts over several years to establish a national journal. M.H. Garvin accepted the editorship reluctantly, but he served in an exemplary manner for nearly two decades. Philippe Hamel, while only briefly editor of the French section, had been instrumental in making the journal truly national. Highly cultured, ethical, and public spirited far above average, he was a force in dentistry for many years, serving the profession in numerous capacities. S.A. Moore, through strenuous efforts, stabilized the finances of the publication at a time when the financing of any project was exceedingly difficult. He was to pilot dentistry through a critical period in the near future.

When Albert E. Webster died a few months later, his obituary was entitled, 'A Prince in Canadian Dentistry has Fallen.' Born at the village of Creemore, Ontario, he graduated from the Chicago College of Dental Surgery in 1893 and the Royal College of Dental Surgeons (Toronto) in 1894. He then attended the Rush Medical College, Chicago, graduating with his medical degree in 1897. For a short time he practised at Collingwood, Ontario, before moving to Toronto. He had been a brilliant student and his ability as a teacher was recognized immediately, and he was appointed to the staff of the Toronto school. In numerous capacities, he served as a teacher of great merit throughout his whole professional life, being dean of the school from 1915 to 1923. Students recognized him as a man who not only taught dentistry but professional life as well. Webster was also a writer of no mean calibre, and his editorials reflect his period well with remarkable portents for the future. He took a particular interest in the development of auxiliary dental personnel. Many honours came to him during his career, including an honorary Doctor of Laws conferred by the University of Toronto. He was the third Canadian dentist so honoured.

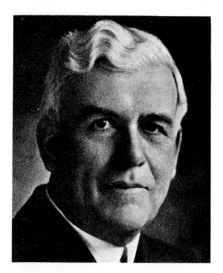

Albert Edward Webster, DDS, MD, LLD,
Dean of the Royal College of Dental
Surgeons, 1915–23, and Editor of the
Dominion Dental Journal, 1901–34

In many respects, this was a time of the parting of the ways. Many of the old stalwarts of the profession had either gone to their reward or were easing their activities; new men were looking fervently to the future. The chief factor in the overall transformation was the change which had taken place in dental education. Recent graduates had received a very different training from that of the older men, and this was reflected in the conduct of dental practice. Of course, there were those dentists who felt that their yesterdays were being torn up and said so, sometimes with more force than logic. But the great majority of older practitioners accepted the new teachings with alacrity, and attendance at scientific meetings increased.

The transition was marked by the recognition given to the builders of the profession by their younger confreres. J.M. Magee and F.A. Godsoe, to take two examples, were honoured by a dinner and presentations at Saint John in 1933. Both men had been active provincially and nationally in the interests of the profession. Magee was the first registered dentist in New Brunswick, and his many contributions to dental literature give us most of the information available about that province during his period. In character he was tolerant, but set a high standard of conduct for himself; mild mannered yet forceful in declaiming principles; genial and kind; a public-spirited man of integrity. F.A. Godsoe was registrar-secretary of the New Brunswick Dental Society for more than forty years. He had graduated from Boston Dental College in 1883 and practised at Saint John throughout his active professional life. Godsoe was a sane, forward-looking man who served his profession extremely well through a difficult period. He celebrated his one hundredth birthday in 1962, at which time he was said to be the only surviving member of the organizational meeting in 1902 of the Canadian Dental Association.

Walter E. Willmott, son of J.B. Willmott, retired from the staff of the Toronto school in 1932 after more than four decades of teaching. He had held some fifteen positions on the staff at different times during his teaching career, while at the same time acting as an official of many organizations. On his retirement, a dinner was held in his honour and a scroll presented. One sentence from it read: 'Following in the footsteps of your illustrious father, who was the founder of dentistry in this province, you have given yourself unstintingly to the task of developing a profession whose members would be learned and efficient, ethical and altruistic, and thus competent to safeguard the health of the public.'[8] After leaving the school, he acted as registrar-secretary of the Royal College of Dental Surgeons of Ontario for eight years and lived until 1951, dying in his eighty-fifth year.

Many other builders were honoured in a similar manner, but the grim reaper had been busy. A.W. Thornton had been forced to resign his position as dean of the McGill school owing to ill health in 1927, and died in 1931. During his deanship the school had made remarkable progress. He was very active within the profession and in many public activities, and a frequent speaker. He was succeeded as dean by A.L. Walsh of Montreal. Walter D. Cowan, founder of the dental profession in the West, died in 1934. Cowan had graduated in 1888 from the Baltimore College of Dental Surgery and took up practice at Regina, then little more than a village in that vast area known as the North West Territories. Immediately he organized the few dentists in the area and sought legislation, which he obtained after a hard struggle. After the organization of the province of Saskatchewan in 1905, he continued as the recognized leader of its dental profession. He served as president of the Canadian Dental Association from 1910 to 1912, and was secretary of the Dominion Dental Council from its formation to 1932. Cowan was a most energetic man serving in many public offices, including the mayoralty of Regina in 1916 and two terms in the House of Commons.

By 1934, the depression clouds were lifting, although exasperatingly slowly. The stresses and strains of the early thirties had brought dentistry new problems. A different conception of the meaning of health service was born. Previously, satisfactory dental service had been provided for some 20 per cent of the population, but now that was no longer considered adequate. Even in the depression economy, those who could not pay had been provided with meagre dental services, and no one doubted that such provision would improve in the future. The profession laid renewed emphasis upon prevention, advocating treatment services for children as the only true approach to improving dental health. Nationwide economic hardship inaugurated discussions, political and otherwise, of new systems to serve the public.

15
Co-ordination
1935-1939

During the latter thirties, two studies were carried out which represented
a beginning of a new outlook with lasting effects upon health services in
Canada. In 1937, the federal government appointed the Rowell-Sirois
Commission to inquire generally into economic matters, with special emphasis upon federal-provincial relations. In its terms of reference, health
services were specifically mentioned. At approximately the same time, a
group of philanthropic citizens underwrote the costs of a national survey
of the distribution of health services, carried out under the direction of
the National Committee for Mental Hygiene (Canada). Both investigations drew upon dental organizations at the national and provincial levels.

The survey report was published in 1939 and represented the first
national examination of health services and public health to be conducted
in Canada.[1] The main activity of the profession had been the furnishing
of statistics, and dentists were rather surprised to find so much consideration given to their services. The factual data were based upon the last
census, taken in 1931. In its conclusions and recommendations, the report
stated that to insure adequate dental services, the number of dentists
would have to increase from 4,039 to 10,362. It also noted that the distribution of health personnel, including dentists, was determined more by
opportunities to gain livelihood than by actual medical needs. Another
significant recommendation for that time was that 'it would be highly
desirable to foster developments in the direction of co-operation plans
for medical nursing, dental and hospital services.' In the context of the
depression, the report was concerned about those who could not pay for
health services and recommended state responsibility for the care of those
dependent upon the state.

Shortly after the appointment of the Rowell-Sirois Commission, the Canadian Dental Association was asked to present a brief for the profession as a whole: the commissioners preferred not to receive separate provincial briefs. A committee on state dentistry had been active since 1928, and the responsibility for preparing the presentation fell upon it, under the chairmanship of John S. Lapp of Toronto. The request for a brief and the date set by the commission for presenting it, May 1938, both fell between meetings of the Association, so that the committee had to work under the handicap of considerable correspondence. However, concurrence with the content was secured from the provincial bodies in time. This brief was the first of a succession of presentations on the subject of health insurance made over the next decade.

After setting forth the objects of the dental profession, the position of dentistry in general health service, and the responsibility of the profession for health, the brief stated, in some detail, the services being rendered for those able to pay; for those able to pay in part; for those unable to provide any dental services for themselves; and for wards of federal and provincial governments.[2] It was frankly stated that the provision of dental services for the whole population was impossible and that 'the solution would seem to be to provide adequate preventive and restorative treatment for the young people of Canada.' The need for intensified dental public health education and for financial support for dental research was emphasized. On the subject of health insurance, the profession said it was 'neither advocating nor opposing any system of compulsory contributory dental health insurance, because of lack of definite information regarding amount of services necesary or the cost of the same.'

Of the recommendations made in the brief, several were eventually implemented, although it took several years and much effort by the profession. Among these were the establishment of divisions on dental health within departments of health, with qualified dentists in charge; support for dental research by government; and government activity in dental health education. It must be kept in mind that this presentation was made at the end of the depression and it was mandatory that some statement be made directly respecting the provision of treatment. The brief recommended that the government assume 'responsibility for the provision of necessary dental treatment for all young people of Canada from age of two to fifteen years inclusive, whose parents cannot provide these services for them.' As later investigation indicated, the profession was by no means aware of the number involved, the amount of services required, or the cost of implementing this recommendation. However, the statement was in keeping with the thinking of the profession at that time.

The report of the Royal Commission was published by the federal government in May 1940.[3] It included a general summary of matters related to health in Canada at that time, with emphasis on the jurisdiction of the federal and provincial governments. Certain statements had direct or indirect effects on the future of the dental profession. The following appeared significant:

It may be confidently predicted that the health activities of governments are indeed only beginning.

The municipality has always been and still is, the basic unit in public health administration.

Certain provinces, and notably Quebec, have taken steps to establish public health units distinct from municipal areas, especially in rural districts.

We cannot see that it would be practicable to assign public health exclusively to the Dominion or to the Provinces.

It must not, of course, be assumed that the Commission is in any way recommending the adoption of health insurance by the provinces.

The last statement was interpreted as being something less than enthusiastic respecting the introduction of health insurance. However, within two years an intensive movement developed for the introduction of some health insurance measures.

The two reports discussed above served to awaken dentists to the need for better co-ordination within the profession in order to meet pressing problems. The leaders of dentistry came to recognize that they must know themselves and their services better, if concerted opinion, based upon reasonable proven fact, was to be presented to the authorities. While decisions had been reached through discussion on various matters as they arose, policy-making had never been a strong point within the professional organizations. And while the organizations had from time to time been concerned with establishing reasonable and adequate fees for services, they had given little consideration to a basis of payment for large masses of people. The economics of dental services was becoming a most important feature, requiring specialized assistance from outside the membership. By the early forties, with added pressures, the leaders fully realized the need for strengthening the organizations representing dentistry. Convincing the rank and file proved arduous and time-consuming.

Towards the end of the thirties, a quiet movement began which was to have great consequences. It started with a small group of dentists who held meetings not directly connected with any organization. All had had experience in various dental associations and societies and sought no personal aggrandizement for themselves or any specific body. They were concerned rather with the lack of cohesion within the profession. Rivalry between societies within a province made the adoption of policy even on the provincial level difficult, and the existing relationship between provincial bodies made national policies almost impossible. Corrective efforts in the past had been based entirely upon considerations of finance and membership. These few dentists decided that the essential ingredient necessary was a proper co-operative spirit within dentistry: if this spirit could be created, financial and other problems would dissolve. From a practical standpoint, so nebulous a program could hardly be considered dynamic. Yet without glamour, without regularly organized meetings (no minutes of early meetings were kept), and without advertisement, the spirit of this small group of well-intentioned men rapidly spread until leading dentists from coast to coast were pressing in the same direction. From this inconspicuous beginning arose a spiritual reorganization of the profession in Canada. And just as surmised in the beginning, practical obstacles fell before it. It would be contrary to the character and attitude of the group that any names be mentioned. Seldom has a movement been so timely. War and other major demands lay immediately ahead and the profession, as a whole, was now in a position to act.

Other long-sought goals were also attained in this period. By the end of the twenties the advertising dentist, who had been a real hindrance to professional progress, was brought under control by amendments to provincial dental acts across Canada. However, some trouble still arose, for the most part of a minor nature, from advertising in Canada by dentists in bordering areas of the United States, where such control did not exist. One such incident, the 'Cowen case,' became notorious on the west coast. Cowen, a dentist in Spokane, Washington, advertised throughout a large area in British Columbia by radio. To counter him, the College of Dental Surgeons of British Columbia gained the co-operation of the Canadian Broadcasting Corporation, then the governing body for broadcasting. When this medium was closed to him, Cowen began an advertising campaign in the local newspapers. Legal action followed. The case was to remain in the various courts for five years. At one stage, a decision was handed down that the provincial dental act applied only to those dentists practising in British Columbia. This decision was appealed. Finally, the case reached the Supreme Court of Canada in 1941. Judgment sustained the amendment to the British Columbia Dental Act which read in part, 'No person not registered under this Act shall within the Province directly or indirectly offer to practise or hold himself out as being qualified or entitled to practise the profession of dentistry ...' The dental boards in all provinces watched anxiously the progress of this case. Its importance lay in the fact that much of the labour over many years in controlling the advertisers could have been lost. The result rang the death knell for the advertising dentist, who had misled the public with his ridiculous claims.

At intervals over the years, a few enthusiasts had discussed formation of an Empire dental organization and in July 1936 a meeting, with this purpose in mind, was held in London, England, arranged by the British Dental Association. The meeting was conveniently timed, preceding the congress of the International Dental Federation at Vienna. Some thirty Canadian dentists attended under the leadership of George L. Cameron, president of the Canadian Dental Association at the time. Representatives from South Africa, New Zealand, Australia, and India were present, and scientific presentations were made by selected delegates. The Canadian delegates once again raised informally the old question of reciprocity of licences, but no progress occurred. The main business part of the meeting was discussion of a basis for the formation of an Empire organization. No definite conclusion was reached. This was the first formal effort, and proved to be the last meeting of the proposed organization.

From its formation in 1902, the committee on military services had been one of the most active committees of the Canadian Dental Association. Despite changes in its personnel over the years, its records show a remarkable continuity of effort through success and disappointment. The achievements during the first world war were a matter of pride and satisfaction to the profession, which worked actively for a peacetime establishment on the same basis. This did in fact prevail on paper for a short period. But by 1920, economic retrenchment was the order of the day with government, and military dentistry reverted to almost prewar conditions. Efforts to alter the situation proved unavailing. The situation brought some caustic observations in the dental periodicals respecting broken promises by government and, in the mid-thirties, a decision to develop, as the only recourse, a sound and detailed plan for military dental services. F.M. Lott, then secretary of the committee, undertook an exhaustive study of all available plans for operation in other countries as well as the Canadian experience. From his analysis, a proposed dental service for the defence forces of Canada was developed in four parts: a dental service for the Active Militia; a similar service for the Permanent Active Militia, Permanent Active Air Force; a service for general mobilization; and the supply and transport of equipment for both peace and war services. This thorough and detailed report was presented and adopted at the Vancouver meeting of the Canadian Dental Association in 1938. By that time, the threat of impending war was gaining strength, and a reorganization of Canadian defence forces was under way. In adopting the report, the Association recommended that it should be brought 'at once through proper officers ... to the notice of the Minister of National Defence'; that 'defence dental services should be directly under the Adjutant General's Department, not under the Director of Medical Services'; and that the 'Association, as officially representing Canadian Dentistry, be allowed to name the Director of Dental Services.' The committee at this time consisted of Ira Hamilton, Ottawa, chairman; J.F. Blair, London; W.G. Trelford, Toronto; E.T. Bourke, Montreal, and F.M. Lott, Toronto. All became members of the Corps with the outbreak of war.

Stephen A. Moore of London had been elected president of the Association and at that time officials served for a two-year period. His was a most active term in carrying out the directives of the Association respecting the creation of a new dental corps. Close contact was maintained with the departmental authorities by the chairman of the committee, Ira Hamilton, and in order to be prepared, Moore himself wrote to each delegate of the Association requesting their recommendations for the position of Director of Dental Services. His action proved most appropriate: while attending a meeting in Halifax, Moore received a telegram requesting his presence in Ottawa the following day. En route, he heard by radio the declaration of war by King George VI. On his arrival at military headquarters in Ottawa, he found that orders-in-council had already been prepared to disband the old Corps and create a new one. He was asked, on behalf of the Association, to name its director. Moore named Frank M. Lott, who had been the overwhelming choice of the delegates. He was also given to understand that the plan submitted by the Association was acceptable in principle to the government. A few days later Lott's appointment was announced as lieutenant-colonel and Director of Dental Services in the new Corps. Thus, according to the records, was established the Canadian Dental Corps, successor to the Canadian Army Dental Corps.

Apparently the initial steps had proceeded in a satisfactory manner. The individual who had drafted the plan of operation for the new Corps had been appointed director, and on his shoulders fell the responsibility for implementation. F.M. Lott had had military experience, as a lieutenant in the First Divisional Signal Company during the first world war. Following demobilization, he became a brilliant student at the Toronto school, graduating in 1923. After a few years of practice he returned to the University of Toronto, becoming professor of prosthetic dentistry in 1931. He pursued research in dentistry intensively and also continued his studies, obtaining his M SC (DENT) in 1934 and his PH D in 1941. The latter was conferred for a thesis on military dentistry. These attributes augured well for the future of the Corps. Many difficulties were to arise, demanding the ingenuity of the best qualified dentist for the position.

No real purpose would be served in attempting to enumerate all the many problems in reorganizing what had become practically a non-existent part of the militia. The necessity of immediate action was not questioned. The expensive lesson of delay which had occurred at the beginning of the first world war was evident enough. The existence of a completely detailed plan of operation at a time of emergency was a real asset. As always, some conflict of opinion existed between civilian and military authorities, but this was to be expected. The greatest single early problem lay in the area of administration. The directive on this point from

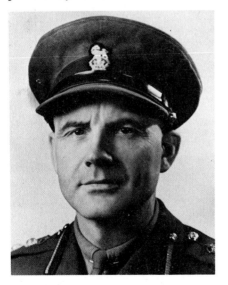

Brigadier Frank Melville Lott, CBE, ED, Director-General Dental Services, Canadian Dental Corps, 1939–46

the profession was explicit. Like all leaders, after his appointment Lott found himself in a position of lonely responsibility. He fought through many administrative battles for an autonomous Corps, directly responsible to the Adjutant General, and to his great credit he finally won out. Once that objective had been accomplished, recruitment to the Corps was greatly facilitated. By the time the war ended in 1945, some 38 per cent of the total number of Canadian dentists were members.

A separate book has been devoted to the formation and activities of the Dental Corps during the war.[1] The launching of a new Corps is a formidable task at any time but to undertake it at the opening of a total war was a frightening undertaking. Equipment and supplies were all but non-existent; organization had to be formed, nationwide, practically from the beginning. All this was accomplished by a newly-created headquarters staff working long hours, seven days a week, in very inadequate quarters, as accommodation was at a great premium. The result of their efforts was that the Corps was ready when needed to accept its commitments with other units of the forces. Of many points respecting the organization of the Corps, one is significant in the light of later developments. From the beginning, the Dental Corps was tri-service – serving army, navy, and air force from a unified base rather than separately. When, after much heated controversy, unification of all Canadian armed forces took place in the 1960s, dentists proudly recalled that they were first in establishing such a service.

Throughout the latter thirties, dental science and technology advanced unabated. Dental organizations gained in strength in dealing with problems primarily caused by the depression. As a matter of fact, many dentists during these years had more time than in periods of greater prosperity to devote to increasing their knowledge, and, as noted earlier, attendance at scientific meetings increased. Improved equipment gave a new appearance to the operating room. Dental units had replaced the old bracket table attached to the wall. X-ray equipment was considered essential to proper practice. Some dentists were even using a stool instead of standing when operating, though this was considered by many as a sign of weakness. The whole range of instruments had undergone refinement, with improvement of the old and development of many others to meet the needs of new techniques. Elastic impression materials were beginning to become available which were to replace the old reliable, plaster of paris. Of all the new materials, perhaps the one most remembered by dentists of the period was the new, lifelike denture base. Over previous years, all kinds of base material had been invented and advocated, from celluloid to glass, but nothing had taken the place of dependable vulcanite. Now the early stage of plastics was at hand. During the thirties, a whole series of products under various trade names became available for use as denture bases. Their natural appearance caused considerable public demand, but performance was not always up to promise. For several years the dentist was subjected to experimentation: each product was recommended in glowing terms, but some warped, others blistered, others distintegrated, and each time the dentist returned to vulcanite with firm decision. By the end of the thirties, however, the acrylic resins finally met the necessary requirements, and gradually took over.

Dean Wallace Seccombe died in January 1936. Practically from the day of his graduation in 1900, he had been a force for progress in dentistry, filling numerous positions with zest and action. By 1908 he was a member of the Ontario Board, and in 1912 he was appointed superintendent of the Toronto school in recognition of his administrative ability. In 1923, he was appointed by the Ontario Board to replace Albert E. Webster as dean of the school. This action was not accepted graciously at the time by a large number of Ontario dentists. Webster was a teacher par

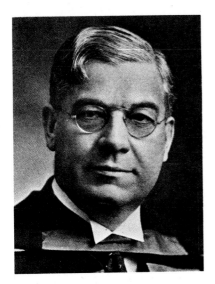

Wallace Seccombe, DDS, Dean of the
Faculty of Dentistry, University of
Toronto, 1923–36

excellence and Seccombe was an administrator of outstanding ability. The appointment occurred at the time when negotiations were under way for the transference of the school from the Board's control to the University of Toronto. Seccombe possessed the type of ability necessary for this change and was largely responsible for the satisfactory establishment of the school as a faculty of the university. His main interests were in dental education, dental research, and dental public health, to all of which he made great contributions. In 1916 he inaugurated the chair of preventive dentistry, said to be the first in any dental school, and served as head of this department until his death. He encouraged the development of dental research in many ways within and without his school. Through his efforts, graduate degrees in dentistry were established at the University of Toronto in 1927. Because of his widely acknowledged reputation, he was appointed chairman of the important curriculum survey of dental schools in the United States and Canada – the report of which was published, after several years of intensive work, just previous to his death. At all times he held a remarkable number of positions within the profession on national, provincial, and local levels. In addition, he established a dental journal, *Oral Health*, in 1911, and served as both editor and publisher as long as he lived. Outside his profession, he was very active in church and community affairs. He was a remarkable leader, a forward-looking educator for his time with an intense pride in his profession. Arnold D.A. Mason was appointed his successor as dean at Toronto.

The latter thirties were remarkable for change in circumstances. The declaration of war in 1939 abruptly altered the environment of the profession. Successful dental services depend greatly upon continuity of service. For economic reasons, patients in great numbers had been forced to be negligent. With improved economic conditions, they endeavoured to make up for this neglect. At the same time, the ranks of practitioners were depleted owing to enlistments for military service; thus the average dentist found himself overwhelmed with demands for his services. This situation was at first considered temporary, but it was to persist for many years, for fundamental economic reasons only in part related to the war. The depression and war years should have been a period when training facilities for dentists increased. The inevitable delay caused many problems for the profession in future years.

16
War years (II)
1940-1944

For five long years, the war dominated the minds of all Canadians. As it progressed, manpower shortages became critical for both military and civilian purposes. With over one-third of Canadian dentists in military service, many areas throughout the country became denuded of dental service. In addition, the health professions became involved in a number of other problems. At a time when both military and civilian dentists were overwhelmed with demands for service, the problems of the profession multiplied.

Health insurance had first become a political issue during the federal election of 1919. Afterwards the issue had arisen before each election, then had disappeared after the voting like many other campaign proposals. Dentists had as a body become rather blasé about the topic. But the depression years had brought forward a great many recommendations by lay organizations for the introduction of some health insurance measure. Pressure developed in several provinces, but British Columbia was the only one which actually endeavoured to introduce such legislation. Amidst much political turmoil, a government had been elected there in 1933 with the promise to implement a program to include medical and hospital services. The medical profession strongly opposed the medical services legislation and it was ultimately dropped; a hospital insurance act was placed on the statute books but was not implemented because of lack of funds. (This act in amended form became operative in 1948.) In response to the general mood, plans for prepaid medical services came into being during the forties, for the most part controlled and operated by the medical profession. Dental services were not part of these voluntary plans: patients who were members were entitled to receive services from a medical practitioner but not from a dentist. Particularly in the field of oral surgery, disputes arose respecting who was entitled to perform the services. It was natural for the patient to obtain all possible services from a medical practitioner in order to benefit to the utmost from his premiums.

The representative dental organizations, national and in most provinces, had set up study groups on health insurance by 1940. The most active group at this time was a committee organized by the Royal College of Dental Surgeons of Ontario. A competent economist was engaged as consultant and a series of booklets were published dealing with the subject, which were distributed to the members of the profession.[1] At the time these studies appeared to some dentists as premature. During the previous decade the politicians had been concerned with medical and hospital services. Comparatively little mention had been made of dental services. Politically, the matter of health insurance appeared quiescent because of the pressures of war. Yet without warning, and with considerable surprise, the Canadian Dental Association received a communication from the federal government in April 1942, announcing the government's intention to introduce a health insurance bill that would include dental services. An advisory committee of the government was prepared to hear a presentation by the officers of the Association on a set date in June. The notice caused considerable consternation because the profession was not prepared to deal satisfactorily with it within the allotted time.

Fortunately, the annual meeting of the Association had been called for May that year. Much of the prepared agenda was discarded, and the time extended in order to deal with the emergency. The studies which had been prepared by the Ontario committee became most important. The outcome was that a set of principles for dental health services (there was steadfast refusal to use the title, principles for health *insurance*) and a draft presentation were prepared and adopted after much travail.[2] The meeting represented the greatest concentrated effort made by the profession up to that time. While many amendments and alterations have since been made to this initial statement as an outcome of further knowledge, the basic ideas remain much the same.

As requested, the officers appeared before the government advisory committee in Ottawa the following month and made the presentation.[3] A revealing point of increasing future significance became recognizable during this hearing. The government committee was made up of eleven men, the chairman being the only one professionally related to health affairs.

The others were chiefly economists. They not only requested statistics but demanded them in the specific form to which they were accustomed. It seemed as if the health economist had been born overnight, and the position of the dental profession was awkward. The president (Arthur L. Walsh of Montreal) and the secretary left that meeting with a distinct feeling that a turning point in health affairs had been reached. Up to this time requested information respecting dentistry had been furnished to various government authorities and generally accepted at face value. Now it became evident that any information submitted would be considered of value only when accompanied by proof in a form acceptable to economists. It became obvious that, if the profession was going to be able to fulfil this requirement, there was need for knowledge which few, if any, dentists possessed.

The sequence of action during the next two years was rapid. In the fall of 1942, the Beveridge Report on social insurance in Great Britain was published and had its influence not only in Canada, but in many other countries. In February 1943, the March Report on social security for Canada was tabled in the House of Commons.[4] A month later, the federal advisory committee published a voluminous report on health insurance.[5] These reports, as well as some minor ones, all included proposals for dental benefits. In the meantime, the profession learned that an enabling bill for national health insurance was being drafted. All this made for feverish activity by professional bodies and numerous appearances before authorities. One of the chief presentations was before the large special committee of the House of Commons on social security, at which time the profession was represented by President A.L. Walsh, Harry S. Thomson, Armand Fortier, and the secretary of the Association.[6]

While the draft bill by no means contained everything desired, through strenuous efforts by the representatives of the profession the content was in line with the presentations that had been made. Whereas the dental benefit was originally to be open to all the population, the bill confined the services to children. In several instances phrases contained in the bill were lifted directly from the principles adopted by the profession. Influenced by the dentists' own emphasis on prevention and control, the economists initially inserted a clause requiring children's attendance for dental care, but this compulsory feature was later deleted.

The dangerous area, and the one where most argument centered, was in the permissive regulations under the proposed legislation. In light of increased knowledge, some of the proposals appear rather ludicrous today.

Perhaps the point is best illustrated by the estimated expenditures. No acceptable statistical information on costs of providing a dental service for children en masse was available. The initial proposal made by the government committee was fifteen cents per child per year. It was said that by some undisclosed method the expenditures for dental services for children across Canada during the previous year had been estimated, and this estimate was divided by the number of Canadian children under sixteen years of age. Through hurried activity, the profession endeavoured to accumulate cost data and after vigorous effort succeeded in getting the cost per child raised to $3.60 a year, but no further. Minimal cost estimates established at the time through surveys carried out by the profession were nearly four times this figure. The experience illustrates that the dental profession was ill-prepared for activity of this nature and that the government possessed little basic knowledge respecting dental services.

Dentists began to realize that there was something more to dental service than practising in an individual office. They also began to understand that covering 20 or 25 per cent of the population adequately was no longer good enough. Lay organizations were demanding that dental service be made available to all the population on an equitable basis. In the past, the professions had determined when, where, and how services would be performed; now the public was demanding a say in these matters. All this led to considerable confusion, and a fear among many members of the profession that untried ways would prove dangerous and costly.

In spite of efforts to fully inform dentists respecting the objectives and critical nature of decisions at hand, the leaders of the profession were often surprised by statements emanating from the rank and file, which illustrated lack of understanding. The position of dentistry was critical at this time. The fact that dentists had recently passed through a severe depression and that the crisis of war was at hand tempered the views of members of the profession. Perhaps the situation was best summarized in a report presented at the 1943 annual meeting of the Canadian Dental Association:[7]

Repeatedly it has been indicated that many dentists believe the institution of health insurance for dentistry to merely mean the setting up of systems of arrangements for the extracting, filling, etc. of greatly increased numbers of teeth. If this interpretation is allowed to remain, if the philosophy of dentistry should be thus determined; then the same position will be ultimately reached by the dental profession in Canada as in some other countries under similar cogent health legislation. Let it be stated emphatically that organized dentistry is *not* supporting legislation to merely set up large scale systems of treatment *but is proposing a definite plan of approach toward the controlling of dental disease in Canada.* The former is retrograde for dentistry, the latter is advance. The first means dormant dentistry, the second militant dentistry; militant against dental disease. The one means making dentists excavators and fillers of teeth; the other places dentists in the scientific and professional health category. A corner is to be turned if health insurance is introduced and the direction taken depends upon whether *a program of control or prevention can be carried through or one of treatment or curative is instituted.* This is the all important matter. Control is possible with an increasingly bright future ahead while a curative program is disastrous and will bog down the dental profession of Canada. *In time of war emergency a dental program for treatment is essential and most appropriate but for an all time peace proposal it would prove disastrous for the profession and the public as well.* The dentists of Canada must be educated to see the proposal in its proper interpretation.

In his presidential address to the Montreal Dental Club in 1943, J.C. Flanagan said: 'By and large, we as dentists have not been particularly interested in that phase of work that had to do with public responsibility of dental health or hygiene. It was a question of laissez-faire and we hoped it would not be a serious problem in our time. Well, it has arrived on our doorstep and ignoring its reality will not help us to evade or solve it. We, as dentists, must of necessity have an internal and external policy.'[8] He went on to say that the profession had looked after its internal policy, but the external relationship was weak and neglected.

These years were critical ones, not only for dentistry but for all health services, and it only remains to relate the end result of the proposed legislation. Health association officials became aware that the proposed bill was printed with all its faulty parts and ready for introduction in the House on 22 June 1944. Representatives of health bodies gathered in Ottawa with concern that day. To their surprise and relief, the prime minister brought in another social security bill, providing for family allowances, the 'baby bonus.' Rumour had it at the time that the prime minister made his choice of social legislation overnight. Whether or not this is true is not known, but in his personal diary for the date, Mackenzie King referred to the struggle within the cabinet respecting the sequence of social reform legislation.[9] This may refer to the two bills known to have been ready for introduction at that time.

This experience had a lasting effect on the activities of the dental profession. One direct result was recognition of the needs of the profession – the need for strengthening the organizations representing dentistry; the need for improved external relations; the need for expert advisers in areas other than dentistry itself; and the need for the development of sound data, particularly in the realm of economics. No longer could the problems of dentistry be dealt with in an adequate manner by the few dentists elected to office: it was necessary to widen the bases of activity. The rank and file of the profession also recognized these needs, with the result that dental organizations gained in strength and stature rapidly. Associations and societies which had confined their activities mainly to scientific matters broadened their scope.

For varying periods of time, there had existed in most provinces what might be termed an oligarchal form of management for professional affairs. This situation existed in British Columbia longer than in any other province. For over twenty-five years, four men, W.J. Lea, W.J. Bruce, R.L. Pallen, and E.C. Jones, made the crucial decisions respecting legislative amendments, rules, regulations, and other matters related to dentistry. Lea was the leader, very capable, determined in effort, inclined to see problems in black and white with no grey areas between. Fortunately, all four were highly ethical and excellent professionally. Their accomplishments were most creditable, but the methods employed often left something to be desired. It became common procedure for them to report to meetings after action had been taken. From the standpoint of the historian, such administration left little in the form of records. In fairness, it should be said that the profession appeared to accept their leadership willingly; but by 1940 the size and scope of the political and other problems facing dentistry had greatly increased. The result was that the membership as a whole became involved.

One explanation why 'oligarchy' persisted so long in British Columbia is that the dentists there were intensively interested in scientific advancement to the exclusion of other matters. Study clubs, which became popular elsewhere as a form of graduate study, developed in profusion on the west coast. Initially, these study clubs concentrated on perfection in the use of gold foil. As time progressed, their subjects of attention became diversified. In a province without a dental school, the development of these clubs made a particularly great contribution to professional advancement. Interest in them continues to the present, but from 1940 onwards a better balance between the scientific and organizational aspects of dentistry came to exist.

By mid-1942, considerable disparity was apparent in the distribution of Canadian health personnel. Enlistment for military service had left large areas almost destitute of civilian health services – and still more military personnel were needed. Furthermore, it was the younger and more active practitioners who had gone into military service. Older practitioners redoubled their efforts in an attempt to cope with the situation, often with disastrous consequences to their own health. For planning purposes, an estimate of the length of the war, which was altered from time to time, became a vital factor. Where possible, the dental course was accelerated in order to produce graduates at an earlier date. For the primary purpose of determining the number of physicians, dentists, and other necessary health personnel available for appointment to the armed forces, and to allot them, the Canadian Medical Procurement and Assignment Board was set up by the federal government. The members of this board were representatives of the health groups concerned. Their first major activity was a detailed survey of all remaining civilian health personnel. From this survey, certain conclusions were drawn. In the case of dentistry, it was determined that 'for the safety of the public, a 30 per cent reduction [in civilian personnel] is all that could be contemplated.'[10] Before the war was over, the percentage was much higher, 38 per cent of the country's graduate dentists. Procurement and Assignment Boards were established in each province, and studies were made of every area to determine the availability of personnel for military purposes together with the essential needs of civilians. A great deal was accomplished but the work was handicapped by a lack of stringent compulsion; politically, conscription has always been a difficult matter in Canada. In some cases, dentists disregarded their assignment to military or civilian service, but in general there was acceptance.

The matter of rank in the Corps became a subject of concern to the profession. Rank structure within the Corps depended upon the rank of the Director-General of Dental Services. At the beginning of the war, the Director was given the rank of lieutenant-colonel; a few weeks later he was promoted to full colonel. In September 1942, formal representation was made by the profession, pointing out the numerical strength of the Corps in comparison with other divisions of the military forces, and requesting the rank of brigadier for its Director. In several interviews with authorities, representatives of the profession supported the presentation. Occasions occur where a private conversation lends more weight than formal efforts, and in the end that was the case in this instance: Arthur L. Walsh, then president of the Canadian Dental Association, and J.N. Blacklock of Montreal finally won the point talking to a senior government official in a private club. Once the rank of the Director was raised, so too could be the ranks of other officers in the Corps.

The first Canadian dentist to lose his life in military service was T.E. Hayhurst of Windsor. He was killed at Dieppe in 1942, while serving as a major with the Essex Scottish Regiment. Before the war was over, fourteen members of the Dental Corps died while in military service.

At the beginning of the war, it was thought that the Corps' need for dental technicians could be supplied by recruiting trained employees of the commercial laboratories. However, this source of personnel proved inadequate. At the request of the government, the Faculty of Dentistry, University of Toronto, instituted a course of training for Corps technicians in May 1941. Members of the teaching staff quickly volunteered their services for the purpose. The Toronto school was selected because of its central location and its laboratories, the largest and best equipped available. Classes of sixty men possessing university entrance requirements were given a six-month course in comprehensive general prosthetic laboratory procedures. A considerable number of these men entered the dental course following the war.

Under war conditions, many situations developed which affected civilian dental service. General regulations seldom allowed for the needs of individual practitioners. Gasoline and automobile tire rationing, for example, restricted the dentist who was attempting to render services in municipalities, miles apart, where the resident dentists were in military service. A critical period occurred when certain imports were curtailed, and among them were dental supplies. Much time and effort was expended in alleviating such difficulties. Throughout the wartime emergency, prices and wages were under rigid government control. Professional fees were excepted, but on several occasions, their control also was discussed. The professions however undertook to control their own fees on a voluntary basis, which with a patriotic motive worked well, and it was the exceptional dentist who advanced his fees without adequate reason during the period of stabilization.

A most humane activity occurred when the bombing of Great Britain was at its worst. Canadian dentists, through their societies and associations, volunteered to care for the children of British dentists for the duration. A number of youngsters crossed the Atlantic and remained until the end of the war.

From the beginning of hostilities, the arrival in Canada of refugee dentists from Europe created a new problem. Previously, extremely few dentists from Europe had emigrated to Canada. Now in a short period there were several hundred. Owing to the shortage of civilian dental personnel and for patriotic reasons, there was considerable pressure for recognition of these refugees. Yet on what basis was this to be done? In making their escape, few were able to bring credentials of any kind with them, and under war conditions it was impossible to secure information from the European institutions from which they claimed to have graduated. Moreover, even if all were *bona fide* graduates, dental education in many European countries bore little comparative relationship to recognized standards on this continent. Language difficulties also had to be overcome. All were sympathetic to these applicants, but recognition could not be granted on a basis of sympathy. A fair and equitable solution to the problem proved difficult. The dental schools set up preliminary examinations to test the academic knowledge of the refugees, and upon the results the applicants were told what further training they required to meet Canadian standards. Through this screening process, a few were found to possess only a little technical training and usually admitted their lack of qualification. The vast majority realized their need for further training and were admitted at some stage of the regular course or to a special course for foreign students. Initially, many of these dentists felt the requirements harsh and too difficult to meet under their desperate conditions, but in the end the same individuals proclaimed the necessity and fairness of their treatment. Many who entered the Canadian profession by this method became most creditable members, and a few have made fine contributions to the advancement of the profession through teaching and research. A point worth noting is that a relatively high percentage of the refugee dentists were women. Comparatively few Canadian women have entered the study of dentistry. Largely owing to the refugee (and later immigrant) dentists, the number of women dentists increased from one per cent of the total in 1939 to 2.3 per cent in 1965.

Problems within the profession arose during the early forties, not directly related to the war, but undoubtedly brought into focus by it. One of these was the use of auxiliaries in dental services, and their proper relationship to the dentist. During the economic depression of the thirties, minimum use was made of dental auxiliaries in dental offices. The war brought a rapid alteration as the number of civilian dentists dropped rapidly and the demand for their services rose. When the depression was at its worst, probably not more than one-third of Canadian dentists employed an assistant in the office. Now practically every dentist wanted an assistant, at a time when personnel of any qualification were all but unavailable.

Pressures grew both without and within the profession for extended use of auxiliary personnel in dental services. The position at the time was summarized in a statement by the secretary in his 1944 report to the Ontario Board: 'Any of the contemplated proposals for change in health services will create new problems in dentistry and alter old ones in abundance. The matter of auxiliary personnel is a most difficult problem for solution. The present inquiries directed toward the finding of economical adjustments of dental practice in order to render services to greater numbers of the population is fertile ground for the splitting up of dental practice. Up to the present in Ontario (likewise in other provinces), a definite line of demarkation has been drawn whereby the dentist renders all necessary services within the oral cavity and the auxiliary personnel performs ancillary services required outside the orifice of the mouth. The specific dividing line has been considered valuable from the legal standpoint. Once the barrier is broken down, it is difficult to know where the next division can be established.'[11] The period was one of advocated change. All kinds of suggestions and recommendations were prevalent, coming from both authoritative and unauthoritative sources and varying from compulsory comprehensive health insurance to intensified methods of private enterprise. From the economic standpoint, emphasis was laid upon the increased use of auxiliary personnel in the rendering of all health services. What happened respecting the relationship between dentists and technicians in the succeeding years may be stated briefly.

The dental technician gained importance in part from his essential role in military dentistry. He reasoned, with some degree of justification, that if a university course of training in his skill was necessary during war, it was also appropriate in peacetime. This point was quickly countered when Canadian universities declared they would have nothing to do with trade school functions, but the need for a training course remained. The second objective of the technicians, who were by this time well organized, was to obtain legislation recognizing their group, and this movement was to go through a most difficult scale of nuances over the following years. Such legislation comes under provincial jurisdiction and, as was to be anticipated, variations occurred from province to province in both proposals and end results. The profession did not oppose legislation for technicians so long as the content did not infringe upon the rights of dentists. In some provinces, joint committees of dentists and technicians were formed for the purpose of arriving at mutually agreeable objectives for legislation. Such procedures in the central and eastern provinces resulted in the adoption of bills acceptable to both dentists and technicians. In the western provinces certain groups of aggressive technicians did not choose to work with the profession, and the issue became extremely political. For over a decade, the dental profession opposed legislation proposed by technicians in these provinces as being not in the best interests of the public. By the end of the fifties, however, legislation was adopted, particularly in Alberta and British Columbia, which infringed upon the recognized rights of the dentist in the area of prosthetic treatment. To representatives of the profession who participated in many heated controversies before legislative bodies, the issue appeared to be decided on questionable claims rather than sound reasoning.

During the years of war, a great number of dentists made sacrifices of time and money in order to serve their profession at a time when their ranks were depleted by military requirements, when those in civilian practice were more than occupied in attempting to meet demands for service, and when recompense of any kind was simply not available. The need was great and the sacrifice was personal. Across the country, dentists accepted key positions and carried out allotted duties, some of which were distasteful to those of independent mind. Under wartime emergency regulations, decisions were made by the central authority, and the most vital activities were initiated on the national level. Repeatedly, meetings were called in Ottawa with notice in hours, not days, with no consideration of office appointments a dentist might have, or any thought given to possible means of transportation, in itself a difficult matter. Those who served without fail under such circumstances asked no credit, advanced the stature of the profession tremendously, and created an unprecedentedly higher level of unity among Canadian dentists.

At the risk of omission, a few of these men must be named in any record of the period. W.W. Woodbury of Halifax, dean at Dalhousie, gave intelligent leadership and his addresses still read well twenty-five years later. Arthur L. Walsh of Montreal, dean of the McGill school, a man of high intellect, saw early the need to strengthen the organizations representing dentistry and worked diligently toward the objective with a marked degree of success. Probably no Canadian dentist gave so much of his time for so many years and so freely to the cause of the profession amidst a practice of high calibre as did Harvey W. Reid of Toronto – a man of ideas, and ideas do have consequences. R.A. Rooney of Edmonton was a focus of strength, no sacrifice being too great when the advancement of dentistry was involved. G.V. Fisk of Toronto chaired several important committees which, in retrospect, elevated the stature of the profession immeasurably. Armand Fortier of Montreal gave strong consistent leadership which contributed greatly to the unification of the profession. These men in particular bore heavy loads of responsibility during the war years, at a time when many decisions had to be made without waiting for normal democratic procedures. Of course there were a host of others, without whose efforts progress would have been impossible. The period was one of stress which brought forth an increased spirit of co-operation among Canadian dentists.

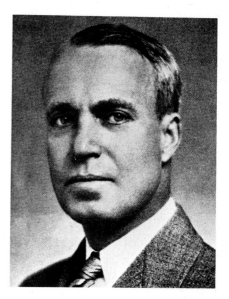

Arthur L. Walsh, DDS, Dean of the Faculty of Dentistry, McGill University, 1927–48

17
Peacetime adjustments
1945-1949

The end of the war in 1945 quickly altered the direction of activity. Canada as a nation was much better prepared for peace than it had been for war in 1939. Gradually, wartime controls were released, and rehabilitation legislation enacted which had considerable influence on dentistry. The most rapid increase of population in Canada's history occurred and was to continue in future years. Many people who had experienced the years following the first world war anticipated a depressed economy, but this did not occur. Demobilization of military forces took place with comparative ease. Members of the Canadian Dental Corps were anxious to return to peacetime practice and retired from military service rapidly. Newfoundland became a province joining Canada in 1949. It was a time of general reorganization during which dentistry grew, and health services received increasing government attention.

Within the federal government, among other adjustments, the Department of Pensions and National Health was divided in 1944 into the Department of Veterans Affairs and the Department of National Health and Welfare. Following the first world war, a Department of Soldiers' Civil Re-establishment had been formed which for the first time seriously involved the government in the provision of dental services for a large group of retired soldiers. After some delay, a dentist, R.B. Sullivan, OBE, had been appointed its director of dental services. Clinics were rapidly established in the larger centres of population and arrangements made for the rendering of services by private practitioners in centres not sufficiently large to warrant government clinics. In 1926, D.D. Wilson, a dentist who had practised at Trenton, Ontario, succeeded Sullivan. The number of clinics gradually diminished to ten by 1930, but a great number of persons were entitled to services which were largely performed by private practitioners. To these numbers were added in 1939 all personnel of the Royal Canadian Mounted Police. An organization therefore existed when hostilities ceased in 1945. But with every member of the military forces entitled to have his mouth rehabilitated under existing legislation, the newly formed Department of Veterans Affairs faced an astronomical problem. The personnel of the military forces amounted to approximately one million; yet by 1949 about two-thirds of them had been dentally rehabilitated, at enormous cost to the country. The number of dental clinics increased rapidly, but a large proportion of the services were rendered by private practitioners. The service by this time was under the direction of L.A. Kilburn, who succeeded Wilson in 1948, and was himself succeeded by Douglas M. Tanner, MBE, in 1963. Both men had served in the Canadian Dental Corps throughout the war.

When the first department of health was established by the federal government in 1919, the profession had endeavoured to have a division on dental health established.[1] During the following years, several presentations were made requesting such action, but no progress occurred. With the establishment of the Department of National Health and Welfare, efforts were renewed and a dental health division was finally established in 1945. The stated purpose of the division was 'to improve dental health in Canada through co-operation with the Provincial Departments of Health, the Canadian Dental Association and its related professional groups, the dental schools, dental research bodies, and all other related organizations.' The first chief of the division was L.V. Janes, OBE, who had served as head of the Corps overseas for most of the war period. He resigned after two years and was replaced by Harry K. Brown, who occupied the position for sixteen years. Brown was exceptionally well qualified. In early life he had taught school for a few years, gained his degree in Arts at the University of Saskatchewan, and then entered dentistry, graduating from the University of Alberta in 1930. He practised in Alberta until the beginning of the war, when he enlisted in the Canadian Dental Corps, retiring at the end of the war with the rank of lieutenant-colonel. Then he entered the course in public health at the University of Toronto, obtaining the diploma (DDPH) in 1946. Under his direction the division became effectively organized. On his retirement in 1963, he was succeeded by R.A. Connor.

No questions arose at the end of the war respecting the need for retaining the Dental Corps, as had occurred after the first world war. The Corps had amply proven its value. Brigadier Lott retired at the end of January 1946, and was succeeded briefly by D.S. Coons. In September E.M. Wansbrough was appointed Director-General of Dental Services, remaining in the position until 1958. On this retirement, K.M. Baird became Director of the Corps, to be succeeded by B.P. Kearney in 1966. The rank of brigadier for the Director has been retained. Effective 15 January 1947, His Majesty The King approved the use of the title 'Royal', and the Corps became the Royal Canadian Dental Corps.

Alterations at the federal level were quickly reflected in the provinces. Whereas before the war the dental profession had one administrator in the federal government and at times his authority appeared questionable, now it had directorates in three departments with satisfactory terms of reference. The magnitude of the influence attendant upon these appointments was realized at the time by few dentists.

The Rehabilitation Act, adopted in mid-war, contained provisions for retired military personnel that were considered generous at the time and probably proved to be more magnanimous than originally anticipated. From the standpoint of the dental profession two of these provisions were of great importance. First, all veterans who desired to obtain educational training were granted substantial financial assistance. As a consequence, the limited facilities for training dentists in Canada were strained to their utmost for several years, preference being given to applicants with military service. Second, all military personnel were entitled to oral rehabilitation upon retirement from the forces. The demand for dental services was such that dentists retiring from the Corps found themselves with an immediate practice made up in the main of other veterans. But difficulties did arise, particularly in the negotiation of adequate fee schedules. An incident which occurred during the drafting of this legislation illustrates some of the problems encountered. During a private interview, the main official in charge of preparing the Act stated that the provision of dental services for retired military personnel would probably cost one or two million dollars. Efforts to persuade him that he should multiply his estimate by at least twenty-five were ineffective until the service had been in operation a full year. Then the profession was requested to justify the cost. A wide disparity of view on the details of dental services often occurred between the government and the profession.

The profession was also concerned about the rehabilitation of its members, many of whom had graduated and gone immediately into the Corps. Preparation began two years before the cessation of hostilities. In every province committees were established which made surveys of locations for practice and stood ready to give advice. A booklet was published and distributed to members of the Corps, containing information about the return to civilian life. This publication contained provisions made by the government as well as the advisory arrangements of the profession. A remarkably generous spirit of co-operation existed during the years following demobilization. In many cases, civilian dentists had undertaken to care for patients of a colleague upon his enlistment, and these patients were advised to return to their original practitioner once he was re-established. Those who were establishing peacetime practice for the first time found other men in the area assisting by referring patients. Local dental societies played the most vital role throughout this period of adjustment. Conditions had altered considerably in municipalities during five years of war. Besides arranging social functions to welcome the return of their confreres, the local bodies tried to assist them with their many problems, of which the greatest perhaps was finding an office. Accommodation was practically non-existent in many municipalities. One outstanding example was the action of the Toronto Academy of Dentistry, which, with the co-operation of dental trade officials, leased a large building and converted it into dental offices. This building became a 'halfway house' between a dentist's retirement from the Corps and his securing of permanent office space. The problems and their solutions varied from municipality to municipality, and the local societies assisted in every possible way.

In memory of dentists who lost their lives during the war, the War Memorial Scholarship Trust Fund was established in 1947. The fund was created through subscriptions by Canadian dentists. The income from it is awarded annually through an essay competition, open to undergraduates of the final year attending Canadian dental schools.

One of the great handicaps under which the profession was serving at this time was the lack of training facilities for dentists. During the war, the capacity of dental schools had been strained in effort to meet emergency needs. Following the war, only a fraction of the qualified applicants could be accepted because of lack of facilities. No expansion of the capacity of dental schools had occurred since 1927, when the Alberta school graduated its first class of seven. During the late thirties, a proposal had been initiated by Dean Mason, and a site selected, for the building of an enlarged school at Toronto, but this effort was negated by wartime restrictions on building. During the early forties, as the ratio of the number of dentists to the population steadily worsened, the profession had studied the position carefully and made representations to authorities at all levels. Before the end of the war, reconstruction bodies were set up and established priorities. In spite of the facts presented by the profession, dental needs appeared to be low on the list of national priorities. In looking back at the efforts during the years immediately following the war, it is interesting to note that neither the authorities nor the profession even dreamed apparently that the population would nearly double in the following twenty years. It was a time of frustrating effort: studies were made; plans were drawn; but no construction occurred. In the end, as shall be related later, the public outcry for dentists proved more effective than any professional pleading in securing expanded teaching facilities.

Another important development which began in the nineteenth century reached fruition in this period. This was the rise of the dental specialist. For a few years before his death in 1900, W. George Beers of Montreal had confined his practice to exodontia, and as a consequence is generally recognized as the first specialist in Canada, although, as stated earlier, R. Hugh Berwick of Montreal had limited his practice to oral surgery at or near the same time.[2] Encouraged by his success, other dentists in the larger cities followed Beers' example and a new trend in dental practice was established. At the turn of the century, the following dentists had confined their practice to one branch of dentistry: Thomas Henderson, Toronto, to exodontia; Andrew J. McDonagh, Toronto, to periodontia; J.B. Morison, Montreal, and Arthur Roberts, Toronto, to orthodontia. Thus the foundation was laid for three dental specialties which have developed vigorously over the years. These early men made a great point of confining their practice wholly to the designated specialty. From this small beginning, the number of dentists confining their practices had gradually increased, influenced greatly by the development of specialties in the United States. The Canadians advanced their knowledge by joining American societies devoted to their respective specialties, and by forming clubs or societies in Canada. Graduate courses also developed, usually conducted by an outstanding member of the specialty concerned. Almost without exception, these dentists were highly respected and specialization developed with little difficulty. It was considered logical, and regulation was in general established voluntarily by custom, although in Alberta the Dental Act was amended, at the request of the profession, to the effect that no person could hold himself out to the public as a specialist without acquiring stated academic standing. In the thirties, under difficult economic conditions, it was natural that specialty practices were affected even more than general practices; and in a few cases, dentists who had been practising as specialists returned to general practice. Some difficulties developed respecting referred patients who had had dental services performed by specialists in addition to those for which they were referred. Such instances led to consideration that the time had arrived when the specialties should be regulated.

The forties brought a surge of interest among young graduates, often before graduation, in entering one of the specialties. In addition a demand for recognition developed among groups other than the three original specialties of orthodontics, dental oral surgery, and periodontics. After holding a series of discussions with the respective specialty groups, the Ontario Board in 1944 adopted a by-law for the recognition and certification of specialties. Doubtless with the experience of the thirties in mind, the groups insisted on a strict limitation of practice to the specialty concerned. The three existing specialties were recognized and academic qualifications established. The requirement that a graduate course of designated length and content be completed at a recognized dental school or institution gave some initial difficulty, but this was overcome by the Faculty of Dentistry of the University of Toronto, which established qualification courses in the respective areas. Thus Ontario became the second province to regulate specialization. The others followed gradually with similar action.

By the end of the 1940s, the number of specialists had increased considerably. Active provincial societies and local organizations of specialists existed, and agitation developed for representation on the national level. The Canadian Dental Association had established a committee on specialization in 1945 with representation of the specialty groups, and in 1950 a group of members applied for recognition as an Orthodontic Section, which was approved. The dental oral surgeons and periodontists applied subsequently and were accepted, thus giving all three major groups of specialists representation on the national level.

The whole subject of specialization has been one of considerable controversy over recent years, and probably will continue to be in future. What is best in the public interest has been the concern of paramount importance. The subject is closely related to the objective of encouraging graduate education. A number of additional specialist groups have ap-

plied for recognition and some have been approved, including prostho-
dontics, endodontics, and paedodontics. An Act to incorporate the Royal
College of Dentists of Canada was enacted by the federal government in
1964, the object being to promote high standards of specialization; to
set up qualifications; to encourage establishment of training programs in
Canadian dental schools; and to provide for recognition and designation
of dentists who possess special qualifications in areas not recognized as
specialties. This legislation was supported by all provincial dental licensing
boards.

The names of those members who established practices in the specialties in the early years stand out prominently in the history of the
profession, as do many of the specialists of later years. The name of Beers
will always stand as one of the founders of dentistry in Canada. Edgar W.
Paul succeeded Thomas Henderson early in the new century as the out-

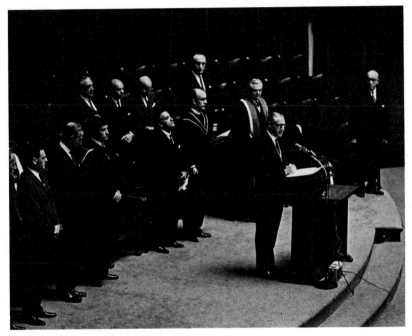

First convocation of the Royal College of Dentists of Canada, Toronto, 1966. The
first president, Frank A. Smith of Vancouver, is speaking.

standing dental oral surgeon at Toronto and took a most active part in all phases of the development of the profession, serving on the staff of the Toronto school for forty years. James Beattie Morison was a leader of merit and a plaque on the wall of the McGill school testifies to his ability. Andrew J. McDonagh was one of the most energetic men in the interests of his profession, the first dentist in Canada to limit his practice to periodontics, and, it is said, the first in the world to hold a teaching chair in periodontology in a dental school (1915). George W. Grieve succeeded Arthur Roberts, becoming an orthodontist with an international reputation; at the time of his death, Canadian orthodontists established the Grieve Memorial Lecture in his honor. These men, and many others who became specialists, retained their interest in the profession as a whole and worked with zeal toward the advancement of Canadian dentistry.

W.W. Woodbury of Halifax was the first to establish a specialty practice (orthodontics) in the Atlantic provinces, in 1919. The first to limit their practices in the western provinces also were orthodontists; although several dentists were well qualified in oral surgery, they did not choose to limit their practice until later. In January 1909 William J. Lea, of Vancouver, announced that in the light of 'the hearty encouragement accorded him by the profession,' he had decided to devote himself 'entirely to the prevention and correction of irregularities of the teeth and to consultation therein.'[3] By 1912, Manley Bowles and Basil Brownlee were established as orthodontists at Winnipeg. These men formed the nucleus of specialization outside Ontario and Quebec. By 1968, slightly over five per cent of Canadian dentists were practising specialties.

Following the experience of 1944, the health insurance question remained in semi-quiescence until 1948, when the prime minister announced in the House of Commons an introductory step towards health insurance.[4] A series of large grants were to be made for specific purposes, stated to be preparatory for a complete health insurance program. The first of these grants was for a survey of all health resources available in the country: committees, in which the health professions participated, were established in each province, and a detailed report was produced in approximately three years. Several other grants were employed by dentistry, including one for public health training and another for support of research. At the time, in a semi-private manner, the leaders of the health professions were informed that the government planned to introduce health insurance step by step, with these original grants to be followed in sequence, approximately five years apart, by additional grants, mainly for diagnostic services, hospital services, medical services, and dental services. This schedule has been followed with considerable exactitude. Hospital insurance legislation was enacted in 1957, and after some delay a measure for medical services was adopted by the federal government in 1966.

Two points need to be understood in respect to health legislation in Canada, which apply more or less to other federated countries. First, under the British North America Act, health matters are interpreted as a provincial responsibility. Second, health is also a federal interest, but Ottawa's enactments are usually in the form of enabling legislation on a cost-sharing basis with the provinces. The provincial legislatures each decide whether or not to accept the enabling legislation. This is a great oversimplification, and much overlapping of health activity has occurred. The crux of the matter lies in financing, for the federal government has unlimited powers of taxation, whereas the provincial legislatures are limited. In the case of the step-by-step federal proposals for health insurance, the provinces readily accepted the arrangements for a detailed survey of health resources and for expansion of health facilities. Hospital insurance was adopted by all provinces with little delay, but the legislation for medical services was a subject of acrimonious political debate, mainly centred around the compulsory and cost features of the legislation. By 1969, however, nearly all the provinces had accepted the proposal. Of the progressive steps outlined in 1948, only the provision of dental services remained.

In the meantime, the profession intensified efforts toward prevention and control of dental disease. Courses on dentistry for children were conducted across Canada, under the leadership of a well-recognized authority, S.A. MacGregor of Toronto. The number of dentists confining their practice to children increased rapidly. The number and distribution of informative booklets and leaflets for public education were greatly increased. Among these was a booklet entitled *A Charter for Dental Health*, stating in simple terms the policy of the profession toward prevention and control, which was widely distributed, especially to all health authorities. These and other efforts had desirable results, for less and less was heard about dental services for all and more was heard about the need to concentrate efforts on the younger sectors of the population.

To the profession, the key to a successful program in dental health lay in its educational aspects. Detailed study of insurance programs adopted in other countries convinced the profession that once overall dental treatment services were introduced, preventive measures 'flew out the window,' owing to the magnitude of the immediate demand for remedial treatment. The need was for a preventive program, carried out by dentists with graduate training in public health. A graduate course in dental public health was established at the University of Toronto in 1945, and later another was founded at l'Université de Montréal.[5] Federal public health training grants became available, positions opened, and were filled by dentists with public health training. By 1950, eight out of ten provincial governments had established divisions on dental health and appointed qualified directors. These appointments augured well for the future: the profession felt that the long struggle for official recognition of the importance of dental health had been achieved. Until the establishment of dental health divisions within the departments of health, progress had depended almost entirely upon the voluntary efforts of dental organizations.

Provincial public health legislation had divided the various provinces into areas or units. Now came an opportunity to test the effectiveness of the policy of prevention and control. The Canadian Red Cross was willing to support financially a pilot test program. A public health area was carefully selected that was both urban and rural and of mixed population, in the Niagara district. S.L. Honey, who possessed a diploma in dental public health, was appointed dental health officer. In essence, under the plan, the dental health officer confined his activities in the area to education of parents and children together with regular inspection of the children's mouths. Treatment was to be performed in the private offices of dentists practising in the area. The objective of the pilot plan was, in the main, to prove what could be accomplished by a properly constructed program of public education by a qualified individual. The results were remarkable. Within two years, the dental health of the children in the area improved by fifty per cent. The project attracted the interest of health authorities, expanded to other areas, and influenced alterations in existing programs. It was a turning point in the emphasis of dental public health. The annual reports of other municipal dental services emphasized the number of extractions and fillings performed for children, in increasing numbers each year. Here was a program which each year reported definite improvement in the children's dental health. The key to success had been shown to lie in direction by a properly trained dental officer. To their credit, a number of dentists returned to university for graduate training and took up positions in the public health field.

In 1938, less than one-quarter of one per cent of all Canadian dentists had been employed on a full-time salaried basis. By 1949, over five per cent were on full-time salary. The increase was moderately rapid, and represented an opening up of opportunities for the graduate dentist. Private practice was no longer his only possible destination. Public health was only one of the areas of expansion. The dental schools were adding to their numbers of full-time teachers; the permanent Dental Corps required recruits; the rehabilitation program of dental services required full-time dentists; the hospitals engaged the services of more dentists; positions in dental research were developing – all indications of the widening scope of dentistry following the war. In addition to the full-time salaried dentists, another two per cent held half-time positions. The change represented progress for the dental profession, but it also reduced the potential number of the private practitioners who were so much in demand.

During the 1940s, also, there developed a strong demand for provision of dental services to welfare recipients. It stemmed from the depression years, when health services were provided for the unemployed, and from subsequent welfare legislation that had been enacted to provide medical and other care for those groups of citizens who were unable to provide for themselves. The extension of dental services to them was gradual, and is still not complete after twenty years. It took various forms in the provinces. Saskatchewan adopted a plan with the administration directly through a government department. The Alberta Dental Association presented a plan to the Alberta government whereby the association administered the plan with the government paying the association an agreed amount per capita for those on the relief rolls; the proposal was adopted in 1947 and has operated to the mutual satisfaction of both the government and the profession since. In the other provinces arrangements have varied between these two systems. One benefit arising from these plans has been the development of statistical data relating to the provision of dental services for specific and sizeable groups of people.

On the evening of 11 December 1944, a large delegation of dentists gathered at the Union Station in Toronto under the leadership of R.G. Ellis (later dean of the Toronto school), who was chairman of the Canadian Dental Association research committee. Their purpose was to keep a long-sought appointment with the National Research Council in Ottawa the following morning. However, this was the night of a record snowfall in Toronto, which disrupted transportation services. The train that was to leave that evening actually left at 5 a.m. the next day after the waiting delegation had stood all night in the crowded station. The appointment was kept in Ottawa at 3 o'clock in the afternoon. The purpose was to seek establishment of an Associate Committee in Dentistry of the National Research Council. The doggedness of the delegation in keeping the appointment despite the difficult conditions did no harm to their presentation, and the request was granted a short time later.

This incident had been preceded by a series of interviews and discussions over several years. For a long time, money had been sought repeatedly for dental research from all possible sources, but the amounts received had been trivial. Opposition was encountered from those who undoubtedly thought that any support granted to dentistry would mean financial loss for their own efforts. Now, financial support became available, but only if two conditions could be met. First, adequate new facilities had to be built, and existing facilities had to be expanded. The universities with dental schools met this problem, particularly the Toronto school which was best equipped for graduate education. The second need was for trained personnel to do research, and this one was more difficult to meet. Capable graduates of fine academic calibre, who were anxious to possess advance training, were available, but no means to support their graduate work financially existed. After due consideration, the Canadian Dental Association established a fund, by means of annual grants, in support of studentships. The arrangement worked well, and with its assistance a considerable number of individuals attended graduate courses in the basic sciences at various universities. A number of them gained high academic standing, forming a nucleus of fully qualified research workers who for the most part joined the staffs of the dental schools.

While these activities did not by any means solve all the problems related to research, a surge forward in this activity occurred. Owing to its size, location, and existing facilities, Toronto initially became the national centre for dental research, but all dental schools participated with gradually increasing momentum. Interest accelerated not only in the profession but also among the public, as a project initiated by C.H.M. Williams of the Toronto faculty illustrates. His plan was organized to meet a crisis in the mid-fifties when several dentists, who had qualified with the assistance of the studentship plan, returned and there was no immediate employment for them. The situation, together with other problems, was discussed with a few prominent businessmen. With resolution they agreed to give assistance, provided Ontario dentists would show comparable concern. A campaign was instituted which raised, in a relatively short time, $100,000 from businessmen and $132,000 from the dental profession.

This fund stabilized the research effort at the University of Toronto during a difficult period.

Efforts to establish dental research on a satisfactory basis had encompassed a period of fifty years. Many dentists had worked ardently to secure facilities and financial support. In the beginning, men like Wallace Seccombe and Andrew McDonagh made valiant attempts and succeeded to a limited extent, but ultimate credit belongs to Harold K. Box who at great sacrifice and with very little financial support over a long period laid the foundation upon which dental research in Canada was built. Today the necessity for research in dentistry is well recognized, but this was not always the case. The rise of a profession to an established and honourable status is a gradual process based on the activities of a succession of men.

By 1950, the dentists of the new province of Newfoundland had become integrated with the Canadian dental profession. Confederation had introduced some new and different problems to the Canadian scene. Newfoundland is a very large island, some 156,000 square miles in area, with a population in 1951 of 360,000 persons served by only seventeen dentists.[6] Outside of the few urban centres, the population was scattered in small villages around the long coastline. Many of these outports could be reached only by boat. Government officials were anxious to secure an immediate increase in the number of dentists. After study the profession pointed out that the primary need was for public education; that care of children should be the first objective; and that time would be required for improvement of dental services. During the next few years, several programs were instituted. Under federal grants, a director of dental health was appointed; with the assistance of the Canadian Red Cross, a boat was equipped to bring dental treatment to the outports; qualified Newfoundland students were assisted in finding places in Canadian dental schools, with financial help from their own provincial government; a program of services for children was established, together with several other efforts. Within ten years, the number of dentists more than doubled. Some difficulty arose when the supply of services ran too far ahead of public education in dental health, particularly in areas where dental services had not previously been available. The Newfoundland experience gave ample proof of the need for public health activity in the improvement of dental health.

Records of the early history of dentistry in Newfoundland are practically non-existent. When John Plimpton came to Charlottetown, PEI, in 1850, he claimed in his advertisement that he had practised in St John's

for ten years. The names of a considerable number of other dentists
appear in old Newfoundland newspaper advertisements; most of them
appear to have been transients. Macallister of Halifax made more or less
regular visits to St John's during the late 1850s. The first legislation for
dentistry was enacted by the Colonial Government in 1893, but the dental
board thus created appears to have been inactive until 1900 when W.S.
Goodwin became the first registered dentist and was issued a licence. The
basic difficulty for a long time was weak legislation. Only in recent years
has the profession in Newfoundland been able to secure strengthening
amendments.

These were years when the horizon of all matters related to health
was greatly widened, not only nationally, but internationally as well. The
World Health Organization was formed in 1948, and Canada took an
active part; in ten years, eighty-eight countries were members and WHO
was the largest of the postwar international bodies. Much earlier, dentistry
had been the first health group (after the Red Cross) to organize internationally. The International Dental Federation was established in 1900
in Paris by a small group of dentists representing Spain, England, Sweden,
the United States, France, Holland, Germany, and Austria. These dentists

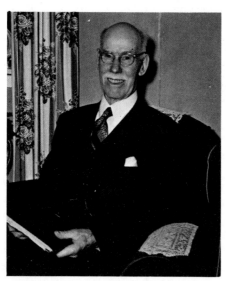

Whitman Smith Goodwin, DDS, first
officially registered dentist in
Newfoundland

had a vision, and it is worth noting the conditions under which they determined to serve. They agreed that they would represent the dental profession without distinction of nationality, and that expenses should be divided equally among individual members. With such idealism, it was natural that dentists in other countries should come forward. C.E. Pearson of Toronto attended the Federation's first formal meeting at Cambridge, England, in 1901. At several succeeding meetings, Eudore Dubeau of Montreal appeared. Except during the two world wars, the International Dental Federation has met regularly since. Following the second world war reorganization became essential, for many of the altruistic dentists from several countries who had supported the organization financially in the past were impoverished and no longer able to assist. During the war, A.E. Rowlett, a past president of the British Dental Association, made several trips to this continent despite the difficulty of transportation to speak before dental societies in the interests of the federation. He was a dentist who devoted his latter years entirely to the advancement of his profession, preaching the importance of rising above local and even national interests to elevate dentistry. In part, it was his influence which brought about the decision of the Canadian profession to take up active membership in the reorganized international body. A more definite influence was the fact that dentists were learning in no uncertain manner from experience that ideas related to their profession were not circumscribed by political boundaries, either provincial or national. The decision has advanced Canadian dentistry on a worldwide basis, and completed its organization on four levels – local, provincial, national, and international.

An event of more than passing interest occurred during the late 1940s, notable because such philanthropic action has been rare in the history of Canadian dentistry. The MacKay family, of Scottish origin, were early settlers in Nova Scotia. A descendant, Gurdon Robert MacKay, left his native area of Shelbourne County to study dentistry at Philadelphia. After graduation, he established a successful practice at Boston, but throughout his life he spent most summer vacations at his native home. On his death in 1945, he left the bulk of his estate to his wife, with instructions that she carry out a plan he had formulated for the establishment of a modest hospital, of which their Shelbourne home was to become the nucleus. Mrs MacKay faithfully carried out the instruction, and on her death three years later left money of her own to supplement the support for the project. The end result was that the MacKay home was converted into a dental clinic, where the children of Shelbourne County receive dental services. Under the terms of the will, the clinic is administered by a board of trustees. It would be difficult to imagine a more appropriate memorial for a member of the dental profession.

In the early hours of 17 September 1949, a disastrous fire broke out in the Great Lakes cruise ship ss *Noronic*, while it was docked in Toronto harbour. In the holocaust 118 persons were trapped and lost their lives. The identification of the victims was difficult, because the intensity of the fire was so great that the bodies were extensively disfigured and partially destroyed. A team of dentists, pathologists, and radiologists, quickly recruited, assisted by the Canadian Red Cross and other organizations, eventually succeeded in identifying all but three. The dental members of the team recorded in detail particulars of natural and artificial teeth which, when compared with charts, x-rays, and other data supplied by the victim's dentists and relatives, made it possible to identify positively approximately half the bodies. Some nineteen had no dental structures. The victims had come to their deaths in Toronto from widely separated areas of the mid-continent. Seldom has a disaster occurred, involving so many victims, when dental records assumed such great value.

Considerable change occurred during the forties in the leadership of the profession. This was particularly true in dental education: new deans were appointed in all five dental schools. H.E. Bulyea, who had piloted the Alberta school from its beginning, retired in 1942 and was succeeded by W. Scott Hamilton. After serving forty years as dean of the school at l'Université de Montréal, Eudore Dubeau retired in 1944 and was succeeded by Ernest Charron. In 1947, W.W. Woodbury retired at Dalhousie and was replaced by J.S. Bagnall (who had served for many years on the staff of that school and for twenty years as part-time secretary of the Canadian Dental Association). The same year, A.D.A. Mason retired as dean of the Toronto school after serving eleven years and was succeeded by R.G. Ellis. A year later A.L. Walsh relinquished the deanship of the McGill school and was succeeded by D.P. Mowry. The deans had served well: their successors could build upon the foundations they had laid.

The years immediately following the war were ones of progressive advancement. The dental profession gained in recognition as a health service. So many people wanted to join that existing dental schools were crowded with students and unable to accept many qualified applicants. A notable improvement occurred in public appreciation of dental health, in large part due to the wartime work of the Dental Corps and the program of dental rehabilitation for veterans. The population of the country was increasing rapidly, and questions related to dental personnel and the distribution of dental services were concerning governments and the professions. It was a time of comparatively rapid change; a time when views of old problems were altered; a time when new ideas were prevalent in abundance. The health services in Canada received more public attention during this period than ever before, and this interest was to prove continuing. Aesculpius had two daughters, Hygeia and Panacea. The first was worshipped as a goddess of health, and the latter has been sought after by all classes of people. Canadians were intensifying the search.

18
Broadened social concepts
1950-1954

Canada by 1950 had emerged from the immediate postwar period and had entered an era when old issues were revived and new proposals made on the political front. The rapid rise of industrialism, the definite trend toward urbanization, the fast increase in population, and the growth of the welfare state were underlying influences on the position of the health professions. Health legislation – rumoured and actually introduced – was considered by dentists the most serious consequence of these trends, and particularly they were fearful of political control of health services. The adage over the years had been that public health was primarily a government responsibility, but treatment services were a professional responsibility. Canadian dentistry had been built by the devotion and sacrifice of a great many members of the profession and political intrusion was considered destructive. The ardour which destroys is seldom mated with the patience that builds. The individualism of the dentist made acceptance of new social concepts difficult.

A whole new field of social science had developed which dentists had great difficulty in understanding. The educative process in dentistry is based upon exact sciences wherein two and two make four at all times, with facts established upon adequate proof. In the dentist's view, social science data never appeared neutral and proof, if present, often seemed based on flimsy foundations. The objective of the profession, to offer improved quality of service to more and more people, was countered by the proposal of the social scientist that the quality of dental services be lowered and spread to more people. The goal of reaching an increasing number of people was common to both groups; the method and the timing were greatly at variance. When reading the writings of the social scientists, the dentist was apt to get the impression that Euclid was not being taught in the schools as well as he used to be, for their angles did not seem to join. And yet a change of attitude was gradually occurring. An increasing social consciousness was noticeable among many dentists, who said that the human story was not reckoned on a mathematical table; that in life irregularities do occur, not abiding by exact formula; and that the element of the unexpected and unforeseeable is what saves humans from falling into the mechanical thraldom of the logicians. The 1950s were a time of intensive arguments at dental meetings. Men do not break lightly with the past. But out of the controversy came new thinking on the profession's role in society.

At no time did the dental profession oppose the adoption of measures to increase dental services to the public, but it adhered strongly to the primacy of methods of prevention and control. The stated objective of the profession was the improvement of the dental health of the nation and not the adoption of a system whereby treatment services would be promised but could not be supplied. In furtherance of this objective, intensified efforts were made to present in every possible manner the prime needs for its achievement. If any program for the improvement of dental health was to succeed, more qualified dentists trained in public health were necessary to carry out the essential education of parents and children. Expansion of both personnel and facilities in dental research was necessary. Above all, more training facilities were needed.

For thirty years, no significant increase in teaching facilities for training dentists had occurred, with the exception of a new school to replace the old one at l'Université de Montréal. The potential number of annual graduates across the country remained essentially the same while the population doubled. Even before the war, the position was recognized as becoming critical. Following the war, the profession pressed for relief at all levels, to both governmental and educational authorities, on every possible occasion. In Ontario, it set up a committee at considerable expense to investigate the situation, but its exhaustive report seemed to have little effect at the time. With the generous financial assistance of the Kellogg Foundation, a conference of representatives of governments, universities, and dentistry in the four western provinces was held in Saskatoon in 1953, but once again while all expressed concern and recommendations were made, no immediate tangible results occurred. While the most extensive university building program up to that time in Canadian history was under way, provision for dental training remained low on the list of priorities.

The records of the profession in the four western provinces show a long history of continuing effort to secure dental schools. Beginning in 1915, practically every year some proposal was made for the establishment of a school at Winnipeg. Saskatchewan had great need for more dentists and repeatedly requested the government to establish a school at the provincial university. The profession in Alberta pressed for expansion of the one and only school in western Canada and gained some increased space in 1948. In British Columbia, most students had for many years been able to attend dental schools in the northwestern United States; but under the postwar pressure for accommodation, these schools quite properly found it necessary to limit acceptance of Canadian applicants. Despite the expansion at Alberta, all Canadian schools were crowded and the accommodation of British Columbia applicants was a particular problem.

In the 1950s, the public became concerned at the lack of dentists. Ill-informed critics laid the blame on the profession, restating the old cliché that dentists were operating a 'closed shop' for their own benefit. After all the efforts that had been made by the profession, such criticism was hard to accept, but it did a great deal to stimulate interest among authorities as to the need for greatly increased numbers of graduates. Finally, an expansion of dental teaching facilities did occur, which will be related in the following chapter.

Distribution of dental services also gained new pertinence. Like other professional men, dentists had tended over many years to establish practice in the more populous areas. When older practitioners in smaller municipalities retired or died, they were not replaced. As a consequence, many people in rural areas which had had one or two dentists found themselves with none. Initially, this situation was considered to be one of supply and demand. Study and some experimentation disclosed, however, that social changes in rural life, together with new ease of transportation and a general drift to urbanization, were complicating factors which made it difficult for any dentist to maintain himself in many of these areas.

Under new pressures, one old battle was finally won. The Dominion Dental Council (latterly named the Dental Council of Canada) had functioned for nearly half a century, holding annual examinations and issuing certificates that were recognized by licencing boards in seven provinces. On many occasions, the Council had made efforts to gain the co-operation of the remaining provincial licencing boards, but without success. British

Columbia did on three occasions agree to accept the certificate, but each time withdrew after a short period; Quebec never did accept the certificate. Walter D. Cowan, secretary of the Council for its first thirty years, and Augustus J. Brett, his successor, both of Regina, worked assiduously in the interests of the Council throughout this half century.

On several occasions, proposals were made to have the council incorporated by federal charter, but this step was always postponed until all the provinces were in full co-operation. Thus it was never achieved. Beginning in the mid-forties, work began on a formula for a national board to which all provincial licencing boards would agree. By a process of revision over six years, the objective was attained. An application, supported by statements of agreement from all provincial licencing boards, was presented to the federal government for the establishment of a National Dental Examining Board. The legislation was passed in 1952, and the newly formed board appointed H.N.B. Beach of Ottawa as its secretary. The directors of the Council, in a most amiable statement praising the accomplishment entailed in establishing the new Board, transferred all records and assets to the new organization.

The recognition of credentials possessed by dentists had been a matter of controversy throughout the history of the Canadian profession. During early times, there had in truth existed adequate reasons for a licensing board to circumscribe its area of jurisdiction, owing to the tremendous variation in academic qualifications which then prevailed. However, as the educative process had become more uniform, there developed a counter-tendency to build fences higher and higher so that it became almost prohibitive for a dentist to transfer from one area to another, even within Canada. The Dominion Dental Council had made an honourable endeavour to rectify the situation, and the prime purpose of creating the National Dental Examining Board was to complete the task.

From the beginning, Canadian dentists have enjoyed and benefitted from a close relationship with the profession in the United States. The development of dentistry in both countries has been along similar lines: the problems have been generally the same, although the solutions have varied at times due to basic differences in law, or what might be called differing philosophical views. Canadian dentists have freely attended professional meetings in the United States and gained greatly therefrom. Many Canadian dentists are graduates of American universities and a considerable number of students from the United States have attended Canadian dental schools. Joint discussions have resulted in the adoption of similar policies, despite differences in implementation. The consequence is that the training and the practice of dentistry are closely parallel on both sides of the 49th parallel.

One example may illustrate the many benefits arising from this co-operation. Discussions were initiated during the latter 1940s to attain common bases for recognition of dental schools in the two countries. The American Dental Association, through its Council on Dental Education, had for many years conducted a survey of dental schools in an accreditation program, which had been successful in raising standards of education and in improving the facilities available. The Canadian Dental Association agreed to institute a similar program, adopted minimum standards for school accreditation in 1948, and through its own Council on Dental Education gained the co-operation of the universities with dental schools and all others concerned. The first survey of the schools was conducted during 1950–1 by a team consisting of A.C. Lewis, an outstanding educationist who was dean of the Ontario College of Education, Toronto; A.L. Walsh of Montreal, retired dean of the McGill school; and Harvey W. Reid of Toronto, representing general practice. After extended visits to each school, the team issued confidential reports of their findings to the president of each university concerned, with a copy to the dean of dentistry. After two years, a second survey was made. Invariably, the recommendations of the team had either been carried out or were under way by the time of its second visit. After it was adopted by the Canadian Dental Association, the American Dental Association accepted the final report of the survey team, and thus dental schools in both countries achieved equivalence in accreditation.

Canadian dentistry was assisted financially by the Kellogg Foundation in initiating the survey of dental schools. This foundation has provided large amounts of money in support of Canadian projects in dentistry, particularly in the field of dental education, and continues to do so. The survey of dental schools has been a continuing activity under the direction of the Council on Dental Education and has been instrumental in bringing real benefits to dental education.

A by-product of the survey program was the growth in each of the dental schools of teacher-training conferences conducted by outstanding educationists. These courses were well attended by the faculty and, by explaining the methodology of teaching, helped improve the instruction offered.

The movement toward the introduction of the dental hygienist into practice began in the United States in 1913. The hygienist's proscribed duties were preventive in nature, with emphasis upon prophylaxis of the teeth. Rather rapidly, training courses were established and laws enacted regulating this new field. Before long, ardent advocates were proposing a parallel development for Canada. Opponents argued just as strongly that only a fully qualified dentist should be permitted to operate in the mouth. After much discussion, the Toronto school established a course in dental nursing in 1919 but limited the activities of the dental nurse to duties outside the mouth, thus delaying for a couple of decades acceptance of the dental hygienist in Ontario.[1] Discussions respecting the introduction of such personnel did occur in several other provinces. In Manitoba, sincere advocates endeavoured at every opportunity over a long period to persuade their confreres, and at least one prominent dentist employed a graduate hygienist in her full capacity until forced to stop by the provincial Board. The idea did not die, however, and with the acute shortage of dental personnel in the forties it was forcibly revived. The dental hygienist's duties complemented the effort for a preventive program in dentistry. The Ontario dental law was amended in 1947 to provide for hygienists, and the first Canadian course of training in this area was announced by the Toronto school in 1951. Similar legislative action followed in the other provinces. By the mid-sixties, all Canadian dental schools either had established courses in dental hygiene or had plans for doing so. By 1967, the ratio of hygienists to dentists had reached approximately one to fifteen. The hygienist, employed in private dental offices and dental public health programs, has become recognized as a valuable auxiliary, rendering services enhanced by capable patient education.[2]

In 1950, the 75th anniversary of dental education in Canada was celebrated at a combined meeting in Toronto of the Canadian Dental Association and the Ontario Dental Association. In speaking of the contribution made by the deans of dental schools, G.V. Fisk said, 'Their vision and foresight have been largely responsible for raising the status of dentistry to its present high professional level. With singular devotion, they have shifted the emphasis of dental teaching from replacement of lost dental organs to the prevention and control of dental diseases.'

The search for preventive means to reduce dental caries had been constant over the years. Various methods had been advocated, and later discarded when proven ineffective through scientific investigation. It had long been established that a large percentage of dental caries could be prevented through dietary control and regular brushing of the teeth. As a result, dentists strongly advocated reduction of carbohydrate intake and strict adherence to effective and frequent brushing. While the slogan that 'a clean tooth never decays' might be questioned scientifically, it was heard in the land for many years.

Dentists observed also that children born and raised in certain areas developed markedly less dental caries than the average. Beginning in the late 1920s, investigation gradually established that the water supply in these areas contained quantities of fluoride salt and that this was the determining factor. By the forties, several large-scale surveys were under way in the United States and Canada. Due to the progressive attitude of the local medical officer of health at Brantford, Ontario, William L. Hutton, an investigation was initiated in 1945 by the Department of National Health in co-operation with the Ontario government. The study began with the addition of sodium fluoride (1 ppm) to the Brantford water supply. It was then widened to Stratford, which had fluoride content already in its water supply, and Sarnia, which had none. The children in these three municipalities were examined regularly over a period of ten years. The study firmly established that the addition of sodium fluoride to the water supply in Brantford reduced the occurrence of dental caries among children by over 60 per cent. This result was corroborated by concurrent studies in the United States.

This new preventive measure was greeted with considerable excitement by the dental profession. At first many dentists thought the results of the investigations appeared almost too good to be true. Pressures developed for the approval of fluoridation of municipal water supplies. Canadian dentists hesitated, however, until the facts were firmly established and sufficient research conducted to prove that the addition of the fluoride salt would be harmless to the community. With incontrovertible evidence at hand, the profession recommended fluoridation of water supplies in 1952. It was followed by other recognized Canadian scientific health organizations. A fact of fundamental importance in public health had been established. But as with all other such measures, from vaccination for smallpox onwards, opponents to the proposal sprang up. Strange pseudo-scientific organizations, never heard of previously, lay groups, and self-proclaimed experts, made spurious charges against fluoridation which were often ridiculous and sometimes based upon fear.

The procedure for introduction of fluoridation has been by plebiscite in each municipality, a method questioned by many authorities on the grounds that the uninformed voter is sometimes swayed by the activities of those who brush aside scientific evidence. As a result of votes, the public health benefit has been lost to a considerable number of municipalities. However, there has been in general steady progress. By the end of 1969, fluoridation had reached 46 per cent of possible coverage of the population served by municipal water supplies (33.4 per cent of the total population). From the clinical standpoint the change has been dramatic, as reported by dentists practising in fluoridated areas. No longer do dentists have to face children with untreatable carious teeth. Fluoridation does not lessen the need for dietary control and proper brushing, but all three methods of control together make the prevention of dental caries at last largely possible.

During the 1950s, clinical practice was revolutionized by the introduction of high-speed equipment. The time required for an operation was greatly reduced and the comfort of the patient enhanced. Many other refinements in instrumentation and equipment also occurred, due to the ingenuity of both dentists and manufacturers. Root canal treatment was by this time a science in itself, and as a result of extensive research periodontics had assumed an increasing part in dental practice. Both the art and science of dentistry progressed considerably, to the benefit of practitioner and patient. The pattern of dental practice had altered considerably. Very few dentists in the fifties performed any technical work in their offices; they had such services executed in dental laboratories. On the other hand, employment of other auxiliary personnel in the dental office increased. The work of the dental assistant was improved, initially by training courses conducted in co-operation with local dental societies and later by formal courses. The dental hygienist also played an increasing role. Greater efficiency enabled the dentist to provide services to more people.

The 1952 meeting of the Canadian Dental Association was held at Vancouver and took the form of a Golden Jubilee celebration. Its emphasis was on the rapidly changing society and the place of the dentist in this new environment. The feeling of the profession at that time is indicated by a few sentences in the report of the meeting: 'The trend of the last decade has been rapidly toward action in the mass. Individualism in many spheres appears to be a disappearing condition of life and with a lack of sense of importance of personal action. The spirit of frustration within the individual is exemplified in casual conversation wherever groups gather together. The tendency is to become dependent upon someone else, to allow leadership to rest on shoulders other than those educated to assume it and to side-step responsibilities even in the organizations which vitally represent us. It is a movement so gradual that it is scarcely recognized and in which the many are becoming shepherded by fewer and fewer. All but forgotten is the fact that the great things of life have originated from ideas and ideas originate with individuals. As representatives of individualism, dentists should alert themselves to this situation.'[3]

In 1950 the University of Alberta honoured one of the stalwarts of Canadian dentistry by conferring the honorary degree of Doctor of Laws upon John W. Clay of Calgary. Clay had come to Canada from England as a child, and had received his early education at Toronto schools. After earning doctorates in dental surgery from both the University of Pennsylvania and the University of Toronto, he had established himself at Calgary in 1906. There he continued to practise for sixty years, while the city grew from little more than a good-sized village to a thriving metropolis. He was elected to practically all the offices the profession had to offer, including presidency of the Canadian Dental Association during a critical period (1926–8).

Matthew H. Garvin also saw the West develop from early days. Like Clay, he graduated from the dental schools at Toronto and Philadelphia. In 1903 he began practising at Winnipeg and remained in active practice for sixty-two years. He was an energetic leader who held many positions in the profession, both in Manitoba and nationally. When the *Journal of the*

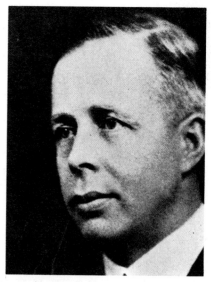

John William Clay, DDS, LLD, President of the Canadian Dental Association, 1926–8

Canadian Dental Association was formed, he became the first editor, occupying the position for eighteen years until 1953. In this bilingual venture he was associated with three French-speaking editors, briefly with Philippe Hamel, then for twelve years with Alcide Thibaudeau, and after 1946 with Gerard de Montigny. He was considered one of the founders of the American Academy of Periodontology, and for a term served as its president. The Western Canada Dental Society established a scholarship in his name at the University of Alberta in 1957; the University of Manitoba conferred the honorary degree of Doctor of Laws on him. It is worthy of note that twenty-one papers by Garvin were published in dental journals outside Canada. Through his own editorial page, he made a great contribution to Canadian dental literature. Other men gave abundantly to the development of dentistry in the West, but Garvin and Clay stand out for their energy over the longest period.

In 1944, Ernest Charron was appointed dean, Faculté de Chirurgie Dentaire, Université de Montréal, after having served on its staff for a long period. Practitioner, teacher, writer, and scholar of note, he took an active part in the progress of dental education and the evolution of organized dentistry. It was not his nature to seek positions of prominence and only accepted them at the earnest behest of his confreres. During his

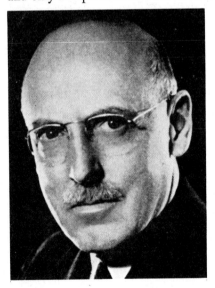

Matthew H. Garvin, DDS, LL D, Editor of the *Journal of the Canadian Dental Association*, 1935–52

fourteen years as dean, he not only advanced his own school to a position of eminence but his vigorous leadership brought about many improvements in Canadian dental education as a whole. Unfortunately, but as he would desire it, his great contribution to his profession is largely unknown, except to the few leaders in dentistry of his day. His quiet advice was eagerly sought, always reliable, and in the best interests of his profession. Illness forced his retirement as dean in 1958; he died in January 1969.

Arnold D.A. Mason, fourth dean of the Toronto school, retired in 1947 and died in 1962. He had served full-time on the staff of the school, since 1927, when he gave up private practice. Because he was himself artistic in temperament, he endeavoured to introduce this characteristic into dental education, which he considered too pragmatic. Like so many Canadian dentists of his time who became prominent, he had graduated from both an American dental school (Chicago School of Dental Surgery) and the University of Toronto. Throughout his career as a leading educator in dental science, he displayed many fine qualities which supplemented and gave poise, dignity, and stature to all his undertakings. No one doubted his sincerity of purpose. He lived by the philosophy that the

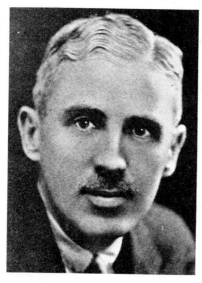 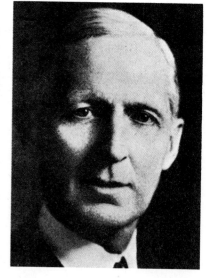

Ernest Charron, DDS, LLD, Doyen, Faculté de chirurgie dentaire, Université de Montréal, 1944–58

Arnold D.A. Mason, DDS, LLD, Dean of the Faculty of Dentistry, University of Toronto, 1936–47 only way to have friends was to be one. His university conferred the honorary degree of Doctor of Laws on him in 1959.

In 1951, the Canadian Society of Dentistry for Children was formed, and gradually chapters were established in the provinces. This action was in accordance with the long-standing policy of Canadian dentistry in emphasizing services for children. Much of the professional and public interest in this area of preventive dentistry had been fostered by the Canadian Dental Hygiene Council. The change in attitude was significant. Once, speaking at a dental meeting in Canada in 1927, C.N. Johnson of Chicago had said that success in dental practice largely depended upon treating children as adults and adults as children. This attitude had been discarded. New leadership demonstrated that the successful practice of dentistry for children was different from that for adults and required specialized knowledge. By the time this new society was formed, the number of dentists confining practice to children had increased considerably; the dental schools had established departments of children's dentistry; and parents were requesting special services for their children. Wisely, the society did not restrict membership to those dentists who practised for children only.

Dentistry in Canada had reached a period of transition. The profession had laboured consistently for many years towards objectives of prevention and control, and now there was general recognition of this sane approach to dental health. Many handicaps existed, however, in the achievement of the final goal. In his address to the annual meeting of the Ontario Dental Association in 1952, Dean R.G. Ellis enumerated the limitations besetting the development and assimilation of preventive procedures. He referred to the existing accumulation of treatment required by the population; the increased demands arising from the social equalizing process, which was creating a much larger group of persons potentially able to bear the cost of needed treatment; the worsening ratio of dentists to overall population; the slow acceptance by the dental profession of auxiliary personnel; the tendency toward the establishment of an all-embracing welfare state; the lag in communication of research findings throughout the profession and in the dental health education of the public; and the low proportion of the dentists' time devoted to the child patient. These questions, stated in a variety of ways in the context of many situations, dominated the thinking of the time.

Canadian dental literature records a considerable number of thoughtful addresses during the fifties respecting the position of the profession.

Among these was the presidential address of C.R. Sellar to the Montreal Dental Club in 1951, portions of which concisely summarize the attitude of many dental leaders in this period.[4]

In the light of our experiences and in view of the many unsolved problems with which dentistry is confronted in the present, our first duty is clearly that of research. It offers one of the greatest opportunities ever given to any profession. Notwithstanding the progress in dentistry, the dental ills of mankind are still almost universal. Their cost in discomfort, deformity, and ill health, is beyond compilation. No one can measure the far-reaching effects of a condition such as this. The problem is one that cannot be solved by present-day methods of practice. Some way will have to be found to check dental disorders at their source. This can be done only by a long-range program of research, it is the public who must support it.

Prevention represents another opportunity. Dental ills, unlike most others to which the human body is heir, create conditions which are not remedied by the usual processes of nature. They bring about conditions that are to a large extent irreparable except by outside interference. It is this situation that has given birth to the art of dentistry, which has now almost reached the acme of perfection. While further progress will doubtless be made in this respect, this is not the road along which dentistry must travel in the future. The art of dentistry must, in increasing measure, give way to preventive dentistry. To a considerable extent this waits on research. Much, however, can be done while waiting for research to catch up with present-day needs.

Dentistry must provide for a wider distribution of dental care among those of our population who are unable to provide for their own needs. In this, the profession should take the initiative. It must not be driven to this course by outside agencies. For its own soul's sake it should assume leadership in any program to expand the boundaries of oral health service. This responsibility, fortunately, is being recognized by our governing bodies, and steps are being taken to meet it. It is the duty of every member of the profession to wholeheartedly support these bodies in this effort.

And lastly, if these things we have been discussing are to be put into operation in the years ahead, they will provide vastly increased opportunities for service. The door of opportunity stands wide open, but as always, only those will be permitted to enter who are willing to pay the price of admission with toil, sacrifice, and service.

In the words of Virgil 'The noblest motive is the public good.'

Dentists, with a very few exceptions, are not politicians. Difficulty was experienced in bridging the wide gap between the utterances of those in public life respecting dental services and the thinking of the profession. The general interest was illustrated when the profession was invited to present a brief on dental health problems to the House of Commons and Senate Committee on Health in 1955. The attendance at the meeting was so great that it appeared as if all the members of the House and Senate were present, not just the committee. After pointing out the lack of training facilities for dental personnel, the representative of dentistry explained that the proper sequence in solving the dental health problem was, first, education, next, research, and then, treatment. Ignorance and lack of understanding was said to be the main cause of dental neglect. Research had already pointed the way to preventive methods, and intensification of effort would undoubtedly diminish the need for reparative services. To be effective, treatment services had to be directed toward control and prevention, hence concentrated on the early ages of the population. This presentation served to clarify the position and created a better understanding in future discussions. Other efforts similar in nature were made at all levels of government across the country.

19

Assessment
1955-1965

Widespread recognition of the country's enormous untapped natural resources attracted increasing amounts of developmental capital from outside Canada during this decade. Tremendous expansion of Canadian industry was accompanied by a corresponding growth in population through increase in the birth rate (23.5 per thousand in 1945 to 28.0 in 1955) and by immigration. Labour and material costs increased rapidly, with inflationary tendencies. As the expenses of practice rose in step with the economy, the dentist found himself with an ever-smaller gap between gross and net income. Dental organizations opened serious and continuing studies of fee schedules.

The relationship of dental services within hospitals had been a matter of concern since the forties. Up to this point, most large hospitals had had a dental service in some form, and in smaller hospitals one or more dentists were recognized as being attached. Generally speaking, the relationship had been casual in nature and considerable variation existed. To a large extent, the hospitals concerned were autonomous, operated by local boards: most government mental hospitals and sanatoria had established a dental service as early as the 1920s. When accreditation of hospitals was introduced, questions arose respecting standardization of dental service. By 1950, when a large proportion of the population was covered by the Blue Cross Plans for hospital care, the costs related to dental services became a critical matter. Further confusion arose around the various prepayment plans for medical services, which also increased rapidly in number and membership, but provided payment for services performed in hospitals by medical practitioners only.

As a result of the federal hospital construction grants of 1948, hospital facilities were greatly expanded all across Canada. During this period the dental profession was called upon to devise plans for dental services in hospitals of varying sizes. Blue Cross officials pointed out the great variation in dental services performed in hospitals from area to area. Through joint meetings, the profession reached agreements respecting types of dental services which required hospital care. In 1957, Ottawa passed enabling legislation for hospital insurance that was adopted by all the provinces, and intensified the need for further clarification of the position of dental services. Hospital legislation is of provincial jurisdiction, and the relevant Acts varied from province to province. Amendments were sought by the profession and gradually obtained, although not without a great deal of time and effort. In the meantime the dental profession adopted its own standards for hospital dental services, and many hospitals have been issued certificates of approval. Conditions of interneship have been delineated and approved in accordance with facilities and training requirements.

In this period, the long continuing effort of the profession to secure increased teaching facilities finally bore results. The first definite action occurred in 1954, when the Ontario government announced financial support for construction of a new school at the University of Toronto. In comparatively rapid sequence, other new schools were announced. By 1968, the number of Canadian dental schools in various stages of development had doubled.

Dalhousie University opened a new school in 1958, which doubled its old capacity. In the same year the first class of dental students was accepted by the University of Manitoba, and a new dental building was opened officially there the following year. The new school at Toronto, occupied in 1959, could accommodate an increase of more than fifty per cent in undergraduate registration, and had ample provision for graduate education and research. The University of British Columbia announced the establishment of a dental faculty in 1962, and accepted its first class of dental students three years later. The Ontario government announced in 1964 the establishment of a dental faculty at the University of Western Ontario, which accepted its first class of dental students in the fall of 1966. In 1965, the Saskatchewan Government announced the establishment of a dental faculty at the University of Saskatchewan, and the first class of students was accepted a year later. L'Université Laval began activity toward establishing a dental faculty in 1968. For the most part, the announcements of these new schools made reference to, and the building plans contained provision for, the education of dental hygienists to be initiated after the undergraduate dental course became stabilized. In the meantime, the McGill, Alberta, and Montreal schools were expanded to accommodate more students.[1]

This unprecedented activity in providing facilities for dental education, while most gratifying, also brought problems. The planned increase in the potential number of graduates per year was over 150 per cent, effective by the mid-1970s. The distribution of facilities had changed for the better: instead of dental schools in only four provinces, there were now schools in seven, at logical centres within reasonable distance of students' homes. But there was a great need for qualified teaching personnel – a need accentuated by the increasing employment of full-time staff. This problem was recognized early in the planning stage of each school, and financial assistance was arranged to provide graduate education for selected potential teachers among local dentists. A considerable number of well-qualified teachers from other countries also have become staff members of Canadian dental schools.

The Canadian Fund for Dental Education was founded in 1962 by the profession. In essence, its purposes are to receive money in aid of dental education, and to grant money for such purposes. This fund has been successful in securing generous support from both the profession and the public. The grants from the fund have contributed extensively to the advancement of dental education.

The expansion of graduate education has reinforced an anomaly. Upon completion of the undergraduate course in dentistry, a student receives a doctorate degree. This has often been discussed within academic confines, for in other disciplines, apart from medicine, the first degree is generally a bachelor's. Long-standing custom has established the doctorate in dentistry and it appears unlikely that any alteration will occur. But for those who go on to graduate studies, a peculiar situation is created. The candidate, who already possesses a doctorate, proceeds to obtain bachelor's, master's, and finally doctoral degrees in his field or area of study. (All dental courses in Canada led to the degree of Doctor of Dental Surgery until recently; but the newer courses at the Universities of Manitoba, British Columbia, and Saskatchewan chose to award the degree of Doctor of Dental Medicine.)[2]

A profession may be likened to an individual. When it is young, it has a strong tendency to emphasize the tangible things of life, but as life lengthens, faith becomes more established in the intangible elements. This attitude is reflected in the various codes of ethics and the amendments thereto adopted by the dental profession. The number of alterations in codes increased considerably during the latter years as the social environment changed.

By the mid-fifties, the great industrial expansion in Canada was beginning to affect the calibre of applicants for the professions. Prospective dental students were attracted to the fields of commerce and industry, where the fruits appeared so bountiful. The problem did not lie so much in the decline in number of applicants as in the lowering of their academic standing. On both the national and provincial levels, the dental profession instituted a continuing recruitment program, to increase the number of suitable applicants for training in dentistry and auxiliary fields, and to stimulate dentists to act positively and aggressively in encouraging young people to seek careers in dentistry. The program took many forms. Attractive dental career booklets were published and the advantages of dentistry as a vocation were pressed through all possible media. The program proved effective in raising the academic level of applicants and in addition augmented public interest in dentistry as a profession.

Voluntary prepayment plans for hospital and medical care arose initially as an outcome of the depression period of the thirties, and grew rapidly. Kindred plans for dental services were subject to continuing discussion at dental meetings but the majority of dentists exhibited hesitancy in developing such arrangements. Early books upon the health insurance movement pointed out that voluntary health service plans became a stepping stone to compulsory measures and some dentists objected on this basis. Others objected to the introduction of a third-party arrangement interfering with the traditional relationship of patient and dentist. On the other hand, there were those dentists who strongly believed that the forces at work in society as a whole made change inevitable, and that the profession needed experience in the operation of such plans in order to establish acceptable data, if for no other reason.

Until the 1940s, the only dental service plans in operation were for school children, operated by municipalities with financial assistance from provincial governments. When legislation was adopted dividing the provinces into health regions, areas, or units, a tendency developed to widen dental plans to include all children within the boundaries of these larger areas. The first of these enlarged plans appeared in 1943 in Quebec, where the government appointed dentists in thirty health units. In 1946,

Saskatchewan established a dental care plan in the Swift Current Health Region, geographicaly a very large area, wherein dentists were employed on a salary basis to care for all children under sixteen years (subsequently lowered to twelve). The plan in Ontario has been related earlier. Other provinces adopted plans, based on health units, which varied all the way from simply providing treatment services to programs of prevention and control.

The first significant plan for prepaid dental services was that negotiated in 1947 between the Alberta Dental Association and the Alberta government for the provision of dental care for welfare recipients. A postpayment plan was initiated by the profession in Saskatchewan in 1955. Several other provinces introduced postpayment plans but none proved to be very successful. More recently a number of insurance companies have issued group policies with dental insurance coverage. The profession in most provinces formed administrative facilities for the operation of prepaid dental service plans; negotiations and discussions were held with a great number of groups, but with little success up to the time this was written. The one exception was in British Columbia, where several groups were participating in a plan sponsored by the profession in 1969.

Like most other countries, Canada shared in the strong social movement which gained increasing strength following the second world war. Perhaps the greatest single objection within the profession to this trend was a fear of interference with the dentist's independence. True, some dentists considered all their own geese as swans, and others were like watermen looking astern while they rowed ahead, but increasing numbers saw that health services were gradually becoming a subject in which all parties expected to help set policy. For twenty years, the dental profession had taken part in continuing negotiation with government authorities. At any one time several matters of concern were under discussion, and difficulty was often experienced in reaching mutually satisfactory conclusions. Basically, the problems of the profession arose from rapidly changing social conditions. In an address while serving as president of the Canadian Dental Association in 1958, A.G. Racey, said: 'How well the public is being served cannot be measured alone by advancements in technical skills but rather by our proficiency in social science and its related subjects.' Recognition of the truth of this statement and others of a similar nature gradually altered the attitude of the profession.

The whole concept of dentistry had widened tremendously, both in the public mind and in that of the dentist himself. In earlier times, the dentist had confined his effort to improving *his* service to *his* patient. Gradually he came to understand that the profession had responsibility for services to the population *as a whole*. The point was one of attitude: the profession had stated on innumerable occasions that its objective was dental health for the nation, but this had long been considered by and large an altruistic goal, admirable but of questionable practicability. During the years of social change, new means of supporting health services had developed, apparently making possible what was formerly considered practically unattainable. The question then became one of method. On this new horizon level a public demand developed for immediate action, alongside full realization by the dental profession that improved dental health depended upon long-term plans of prevention and control.

In 1961, the federal government appointed a Royal Commission on Health Services. During the following two years, this commission held hearings at strategic centres across Canada. Briefs were presented in great numbers by both professional and lay groups. Some twenty organizations representing the dental profession made presentations which dealt in detail with dental health services and laid down a definite plan of procedure directed toward improved national dental health. Many of the presentations by lay groups were extreme in their demands – so much so that at one hearing a member of the commission was moved to state that no matter what was recommended, government legislation could not provide for the establishment of health services in the front yard of every farmhouse.

In an extensive and well-documented brief, the Canadian Dental Association pointed out that the dental health problem would never be solved unless the prevalence and incidence of dental diseases were decreased; that the economic factor was not the only or even the most important cause of poor dental health; that the Association could *not* recommend a national dental health insurance plan under existing circumstances; that if the commission should nevertheless recommend the establishment of a dental insurance plan, it should be preceded by and accompanied by intensive dental health education and confined to the youngest age groups of the population, with annual extension to children one year older. The specific recommendations made in the brief are summarized in Appendix K. The goal of the dental profession was stated as the improvement of the level of dental health until ultimately all Canadians enjoyed good dental health.

The presentation was well received by both the commission and the press. This submission, together with the briefs from all other dental organizations, represented the greatest effort ever made to that date by the dental profession to present the factors related to dental health in Canada. Their effectiveness was found in the report of the commission.

The Royal Commission issued a voluminous report which contained an unprecedented number of recommendations respecting dentistry.[3] After pointing to the 'paradox of our age' as being 'the enormous gap between scientific knowledge and skills on one hand, and our organizations and financial arrangements to apply them to the needs of men, on the other,' the commission recommended 'a comprehensive universal health services program for the Canadian people.' The majority of the recommendations respecting dental services were for the most part in accordance with the proposals made by the profession. These included support for fluoridation of community water supplies, dental health educational programs, increased funds for dental research, dental treatment benefits for all beneficiaries under public assistance programs, immediate action in increasing teaching facilities, hospital arrangements for dental services, and several other points. In agreement with the dental profession, the commission stated that the approach to dental health should begin with the youngest age groups of the population. Contrary to the proposals of the profession, it also recommended, in considerable detail, the establishment of dental clinics as the method of implementing the children's program, and further, that dental auxiliaries be trained 'to prepare cavities and place fillings in the teeth of children and undertake dental health education and give instruction to patients in self care.' The report stated that 'This program must have one of the highest priorities among our proposals.' The dental profession reacted strongly against this method of dealing with dental care for the age groups that are most important from the standpoint of control and prevention.

If a profession is to develop into a scientific body, there must be leaders who adhere strongly to the principles underlying this objective. The price must be paid. Canadian dentistry has been fortunate in its leadership and the names of many of these men have appeared in this book. For over forty years, Sydney W. Bradley of Ottawa laboured consistently toward stabilizing the scientific foundation of dentistry. All through his life, he quietly and without publicity gave support to a remarkable number of projects designed to this end. One of the conditions attached to his contributions was strict privacy. He was an astute man in the financial world. While he was elected to many professional offices and honoured in several ways, his main contribution consisted of financial assistance: no other Canadian dentist gave so much of his worldly possessions to his profession. During his later years, he evolved the idea that a national library was an essential part of any scientific profession. Such a library was established in 1951 at the headquarters of the national association, and he consistently gave support in large amounts on an annual basis to its development, without the knowledge of his confreres. When he died in 1967, his will left money to assist in the maintenance of the library, which was then named the Sydney Wood Bradley Memorial Library.

From the earliest times, Canadian dentists have been very active in public life, particularly on the municipal level, and have occupied positions of trust in many capacities. J.B. Willmott was Justice of the Peace in the town of Milton before coming to Toronto. One of the early dentists of Montreal, Aldis Bernard, became mayor of that city in 1873 after an active career in city affairs. Throughout the years, dentists in great number have served municipal, educational, and charitable institutions with distinction. A considerable number have been elected to their provincial legislatures, and a few have served as members of the federal Parliament, beginning with W.D. Cowan of Regina in 1917.[4] Comparatively few dentists have left the ranks of their profession to enter other vocations. A notable exception however was Gaspard Fauteux, who while serving as a member of the House of Commons became Speaker of the House, and was created a member of the Privy Council in 1949. He then became Lieutenant-Governor of his native province of Quebec, serving from 1950 to 1958.

The percentage of women dentists in Canada is low when compared to several other countries. Probably the prime reason why more women do not enter the study of dentistry is established custom. Only in recent years have many Canadian women after marriage engaged in vocations as a life pursuit. Another deterrent may be the cost of dental education, one of the highest among the professions. The number of women graduates in most professions in Canada is not high, although higher in medicine than in dentistry.[5] With the strong emphasis on children's dentistry, there has developed a real opportunity for more women dentists; and those who are in practice invariably have excellent clienteles and report incomes comparable to the men. The profession has endeavoured to attract women to dentistry, believing that services to the public would benefit, but with little apparent result to date.

In early times, the dentist was forced to invent his own instruments and equipment, if he was to have any. Many of the operative tools used today are improved models of those originally designed by early dentists. As time passed and new techniques developed, the instruments and materials became further improved through research by manufacturers of dental supplies. However, dentists also continued to design instruments and equipment to meet their needs. Some dentists did not confine their inventive efforts to devices related to dentistry. Even a casual examination of patent listings reveals the names of a great number of members of the dental profession. The basic patent on the rotary snowplow for railway locomotives was taken out by J.W. Elliott, a Toronto dentist, in 1869. He appears to have been one of the first dentists to invent a practical device to meet a real need: his design is still employed in the snowblowers many

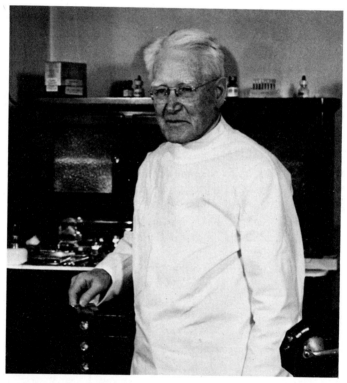

E.R.K. Hart established his practice at Sackville, NB, in 1898. At the age of 95 in 1969, he was still practising in the original office, stating that he had no intention of retiring or of cutting down on his work week.

householders use today. Throughout the years, other inventive dentists have been active in the areas of gas-burning, magnetic, and electrical devices. Like inventors in general, many have gained no financial advantage but some have done well economically through royalties.[6]

The literary production of Canadian dentists has not been abundant, although many papers published in professional journals exhibit marked ability. It may seem surprising, but dentists have published more poetry than prose. A few poems written by Dean Thornton of McGill have survived and show talent; Mark McElhinney of Ottawa published a book of poems in 1927; W.A. Black of Toronto wrote considerable poetry, some of which appeared in dental journals; I.B. Ezra of Windsor published a book of poetry in 1951; several poems of literary merit were published by Joseph Nolin of Montreal; and others have published lesser amounts of poetry. In prose, George Frederick Clarke of Woodstock, NB, is by far the most outstanding of Canadian dentists.[7] During his lifetime, he has published some fifteen books and sixty stories and articles, one of the books in 1968 when he was eighty-five years old. His writings have enjoyed a worldwide distribution. Also from New Brunswick, at an earlier date, F.K. Crosby published a considerable amount, chiefly in prominent magazines of the United States. He was a highly cultured man and his publications are probably second in quantity only to Clarke's. A few other dentists have written literature of merit but in general production has been meagre.

No statement appears more continuously or frequently in dental literature than the one that dentistry is both an art and a science. Basic dictionary meanings of 'art' as 'skill' and 'science' as 'of knowledge,' meaning knowledge of the basic sciences, in one sense furnish a measuring stick for the advancement of the profession. Dentistry began as a skill, and science gradually became an integral part, developing very rapidly after the turn of the century. The scientific education of the dentist today has little in common with that of the graduate of a few decades ago. At some stage of development a balance was reached, between art and science, making a true health profession. The speculative student of the history of dentistry finds great difficulty in establishing an exact date when this occurred. He may even be inclined to conclude that the relationship is an ever-changing one.

Historically, Canadian dentistry advanced very rapidly from skill to scientific profession. The early difficulties in gaining recognition of dental care as an essential health need have long since been overcome. The long struggle for adequate teaching facilities and qualified educational personnel is largely over. The long-standing policies of the dental profession respecting prevention and control of dental diseases have become recognized by authorities. Dental research receives increasing financial support. These and many other factors augur well for the future.

After years of stringent labour, a solid foundation for the profession has been established. Objectives, which were initially considered altruistic by many, have become recognized as reality through the ardent advocacy of a host of humane dentists. To these men, the dental profession owes all that Canadian dentistry stands for today. The progress of the past is the encouragement for the future. No viable profession can afford to clip the coupons of the history of its past and take it all for granted. The task of the historian is to relate the past, with explanation, and not to predict the future.

Within the last 15 years, the facilities for training new dentists in Canada have more than doubled to meet growing national demands for oral health services. New faculties have been opened in five provinces; established schools have been enlarged and modernized. On the next four pages is a sampling of scenes of modern dental education, spanning the country from Pacific to Atlantic.

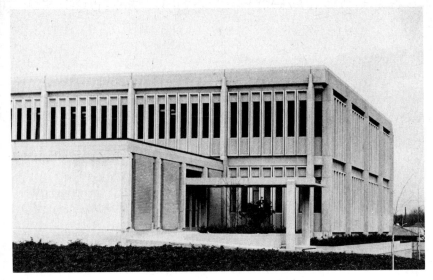

Dental Building, University of British Columbia, opened in 1968

Oral pathology laboratory, University of Alberta

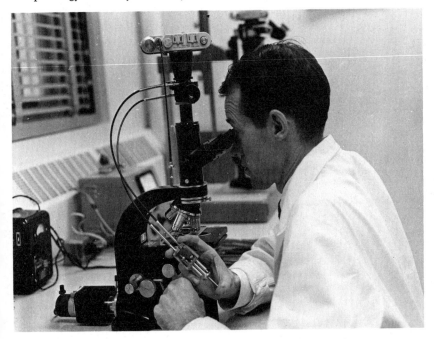

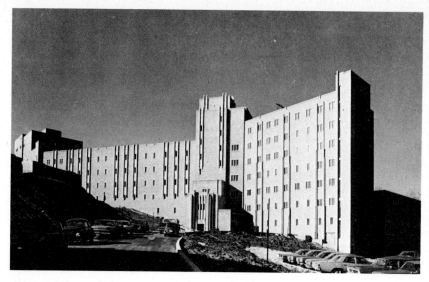

Health Sciences Building, University of Western Ontario. The Faculty of Dentistry is one occupant of this major new complex, completed in 1968

Dental materials research laboratory, University of Manitoba

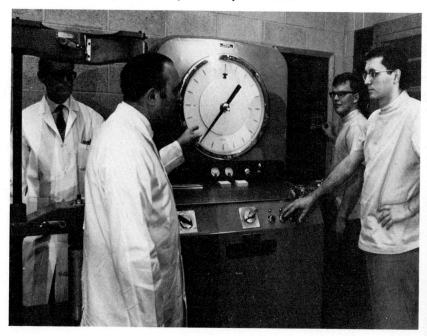

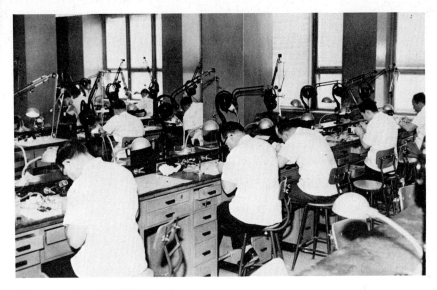

Laboratory class, McGill University

Closed circuit TV has become a major teaching tool in dentistry. Students at their lectures can see the same close-up of the patient's mouth as appears on the monitor in this University of Toronto studio

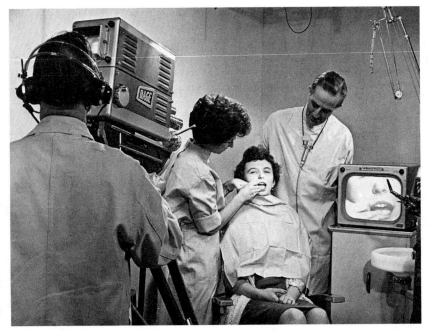

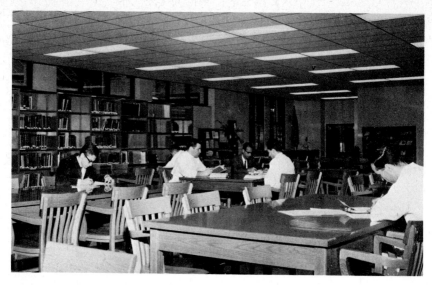

Dental library, Université de Montréal

Dentists-to-be practise their science in the clinic at Dalhousie University, opened in 1958

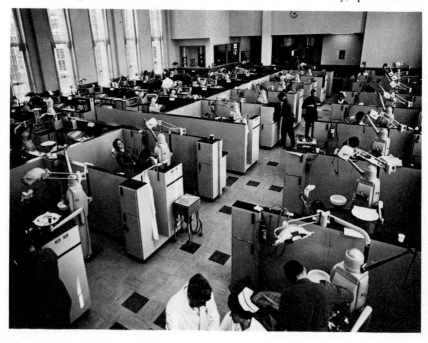

Notes

CHAPTER 1 *Pages 3–10*

1 J.E. Anderson, 'The People of Fairty,' *Contributions to Anthropology 1961–2*, Part 1, National Museum of Canada Bulletin No 193
2 J.E. Anderson, 'A Pre-Iroquois Burial Site,' *Ontario Archaeology*, Publication No 7, the Ontario Archaeological Society, 1962
3 Kenneth E. Kidd, 'The Excavation and Historical Identification of a Huron Ossuary,' *American Antiquity*, Vol 18
4 Anderson, 'A Pre-Iroquois Burial Site'
5 Edith VanAllen Murphy, *Indian Uses of the Native Plants* (Desert Printers, Palm Desert, California, 1959)
6 Percy W. Mathews, 'Notes on Diseases among the Indians Frequenting York Factory, Hudson Bay,' *Canada Medical and Surgical Journal*, Vol 13, 1885
7 J.C. Boileau Grant, *Anthropology of the Chipewayan and Cree Indians*, National Museum of Canada Bulletin No 64, Anthropological Series No 14, 1930
8 Personal communication from James Tuck, Department of Sociology and Anthropology, Memorial University, St. John's, Newfoundland
9 'Discovery of prehistoric cemetery reveals Ohio Indians with arthritis and bad teeth,' *Journal of the American Dental Association*, 1968
10 C.H.M. Williams, 'An Investigation concerning the Dentition of Eskimos of Canada's Eastern Arctic,' *Journal of American Academy of Periodontology*, 1942
11 D. Jenness, *Indians of Canada* (Ottawa, 1932)
12 See the article by A. de H. Smith, *Dominion Dental Journal*, Vol 34, December 1922.
13 H.P. Biggar, *Voyages of Jacques Cartier*, Public Archives of Canada Bulletin No 11, 1924
14 N.E. Dionne, *Champlain* (Toronto, 1905)
15 Norah Storey, *The Oxford Companion to Canadian History and Literature* (Toronto, 1967)
16 Fielding H. Garrison, *An Introduction to the History of Medicine* (Toronto, 1929)

17 Maude E. Abbott, *History of Medicine in the Province of Quebec* (Montreal, 1931). See also *Dictionary of Canadian Biography*, Vol I (Toronto, 1966)
18 *Almanach de Québec pour l'anné 1791* (Quebec Public Archives)

CHAPTER 2   *Pages 11–20*

1 Communication to author from Department of Northern Affairs
2 Menzies Campbell, *From a Trade to a Profession* (published for private circulation, 1958)
3 *Dominion Dental Journal*, Vol 26, No 6, June 1914
4 *The Examiner*, Toronto, 1 January 1840
5 Printed by R. Stanton, who was publisher of the *Upper Canada Gazette*, Printer to the King's Most Excellent Majesty, general printer, stationer, and bookbinder at 164 King Street West, Toronto, over a considerable number of years.
6 W.H. Graham, *The Tiger of Canada West* (Toronto, 1962)
7 E.C. Guillet, *The Pioneer Farmer and Backwoodsman* (Toronto, 1963)
8 *Ibid.*
9 *The Telegram*, Toronto, 24 December 1933

CHAPTER 3   *Pages 21–38*

1 Montreal Judicial Archives
2 Nova Scotia Public Archives, Halifax
3 A.J. McAvenney, 'Early History of Dentistry in New Brunswick,' *Dominion Dental Journal*, Vol 17, December 1905
4 The first foot engine was invented by Morrison in 1872.
5 J.A. Bazin, 'Yesterday,' *Dominion Dental Journal*, Vol 4, May 1892
6 Descriptions of the key are to be found in numerous books on the history of dentistry. One of the best concise accounts of the development and use of this instrument is in the Catalogue of the Menzies Campbell Collection, prepared by J. Menzies Campbell (Royal College of Surgeons of Edinburgh, 1966).
7 Annual reports of this dispensary in the Nova Scotia Public Archives show considerable dental services rendered each year. The report for 1891 points to 'benefits derived from substituting for indiscriminating extraction that of preservative treatment,' The dispensary continued to operate until the 1920s when it was replaced by school dental clinics.
8 *Northwest Digest*, 19 June 1858
9 *Victoria Gazette*, 23 June 1859
10 Trade licenses assessment lists, Victoria, 1863
11 See Appendix A, Dentists of 1858.
12 A complete file of *The Nor'wester* is in the Manitoba Public Archives, Winnipeg.
13 *Bulletin des recherches historiques*, Vol 41 and 49
14 Quebec Public Archives
15 *Dominion Dental Journal*, January 1890

CHAPTER 4   *Pages 39–54*

1 No copy of this circular letter has been found but a description of its contents by Day appears in the *Dominion Dental Journal*, Vol 10, p 354. Its content is also stated by several others in the literature.

2 W. George Beers, 'Sketch of Dentistry in Canada,' *Dominion Dental Journal* Vol 12, July 1900

3 Robert M. Warner, *Profile of a Profession: A History of the Michigan State Dental Association* (Detroit, 1964)

4 The copy of this first constitution and bylaws was lost for a long period, and was found among the papers of J. Neelands. It was then published in the *Dominion Dental Journal*, Vol 39, p 171.

5 The *Globe* reported the meeting at some length, featuring the fact that the organizers were from 'east of Port Hope.'

6 See Appendix B, Petition to the Ontario Legislature, 1868.

7 See Appendix C, The World's First Dental Act.

8 Private communication with the author

9 The use of the term 'Royal' in the legislation establishing the Royal College of Dental Surgeons of Ontario in 1868 has been somewhat of a mystery, subject of speculation over the years. Of the provincial professional acts, this is the only one in which the term appears in the title of the body established. Such use of 'Royal' requires permission of the Queen, a matter requiring considerable time: it must first have the sanction of the Secretary of State, who passes the request, if approved, on to the Governor-General, who if in agreement in turn forwards the request to Buckingham Palace for permission. Even with modern means of communication, this procedure is likely to require a minimum of six months and probably longer. In 1868, the Ontario dental bill was introduced on January 30 and passed on March 3. Preceding introduction some action may have occurred respecting the title, but this could not have happened before late 1867, because the preliminary draft was not prepared until near the end of that year. Diligent search for an answer to this mystery has been made without result. Authorities state that the word 'Royal' would not appear in such legislation without permission. The papers of John Sandfield Macdonald, first premier of Ontario, are largely lost, but the remaining ones are deposited at the Public Archives of Canada, Ottawa. Search of these papers has revealed no reference to the matter. These archives possess an accurate list of permissions granted for the use of the term 'Royal' but this list dates only from 1889.

10 A.J. McAvenney, 'Early History of Dentistry in New Brunswick,' *Dominion Dental Journal*, Vol 17, November 1905

11 W. George Beers, 'Poor Nova Scotia,' *Canadian Journal of Dental Science*, Vol 3, March 1871

12 In a private letter to the author, John J. Salley, Dean of the School of Dentistry, University of Maryland, states: 'Professor Foley further advises that the first and only Canadian dentist to receive an honorary degree (from the Baltimore College of Dental Surgery) was a Dr J. Fayne in 1847. Another Canadian dentist, Dr E.P. Burroughs, was graduated in 1846. This would make Dr Burroughs the first Canadian graduate instead of Dr Nelles. Our records show that Dr Burroughs was the first graduate from a country outside the United States.' Diligent search has not resulted in finding either of these names among Canadian dentists. Presumably they may not have returned to Canada to practice.

13 No copies of *The Family Dentist* have been found. The *Journal of the Times* was a letterhead-size, four-page quarterly, of which seven issues were published in total. Perusal of the issues shows that only the first page was devoted to dental subjects. The other pages contained a miscellany of short items and verses of a general nature, extracted from various publications and dealing with subjects from philosophy to odd news events, interspersed with statements respecting the dental practice of Macallister and Paine of an advertising nature. A few adver-

tisements by merchants appeared. Evidently a thief had stolen the street sign of the publishers' office, for the following notice appeared in the second issue:

THE SIGN OF THE GOLDEN TOOTH

If the person or persons who a few weeks ago stole the large golden tooth from over our door, (we suppose they must have thought it was solid gold) finding it worthless, at least to themselves, will return it, we will not only suitably reward them for their trouble, but will extract all their teeth without charge. This was the largest tooth ever extracted and was originally removed from the mouth of the Kennebeck River; and its loss has caused our cheeks to fall in very much. If the tooth is not returned to us soon, we shall have to supply its loss by an artificial tooth of our own manufacture.

There is no indication in the next following issues that the tooth was returned.

14 Henry T. Wood, 'Dentistry and Dentists in Ontario before 1868,' *Dominion Dental Journal*, Vol 10, July 1898

15 *Canada Medical Journal*, Vol 7, 1870–1

16 W. George Beers, 'Amalgam for Filling Teeth,' *Canada Journal of Dental Science*, Vol 3, April 1871

CHAPTER 5   *Pages 55–65*

1 *Canada Journal of Dental Science*, Vol 3, May 1871
2 Minutes of the Royal College of Dental Surgeons of Ontario, July 1871
3 *Canada Journal of Dental Science*, Vol 3, June 1871
4 *Ibid.*
5 *Canada Journal of Dental Science*, Vol 3, December 1870
6 Minutes of the Royal College of Dental Surgeons of Ontario, July 1875
7 *Ibid.*
8 The name of the school used in the text is 'Royal College of Dental Surgeons' or 'Toronto school.' The annual announcements of the school from the first (see page 59) up to 1904 bore the title, 'The School of Dentistry, Toronto.' No reference to a change of name has been found in the official records, but from 1905 to 1924 the name used in announcements was 'Royal College of Dental Surgeons of Ontario in affiliation with the University of Toronto.' From 1925 onwards, the name used has been, 'Faculty of Dentistry, University of Toronto.' But when the school was built at College and Huron Streets in 1909, 'Royal College of Dental Surgeons' was cut in large letters in the stone above the front door, and references to the school contained in records relating to the transfer of the school to the University of Toronto used the name, 'Royal College of Dental Surgeons.'
9 Minutes of the Royal College of Dental Surgeons of Ontario, January 1877
10 *Canada Journal of Dental Science*, Vol 4, November 1877
11 *Canada Journal of Dental Science*, Vol 4, March 1878
12 *Canada Journal of Dental Science*, Vol 3, December 1870
13 *Canada Journal of Dental Science*, Vol 2, August 1870

CHAPTER 6   *Pages 66–80*

1 Information respecting F.D. Shaw and William Wilson is courtesy of the Glenbow-Alberta Institute, Calgary.
2 Personal communication to the author
3 Tony Cashman, 'Edmonton Story,' *The Edmontonian*
4 *British Columbia Gazette,* 16 January 1890

5 Nova Scotia Public Archives
6 In view of the statement on this point made in the preceding chapter, some explanation is necessary. The actual motion adopted by the Board of the Royal College of Dental Surgeons of Ontario on 31 March 1893 reads: 'That J.B. Willmott be, and is hereby appointed dean of the school of dentistry at a salary of $250.00 per annum.' This is the first official action recorded in the minutes respecting the position of dean. The announcement referred to was issued for the year 1888–9. Willmott had been regularly referred to in the dental literature as dean. Two minor references are contained in the Board minutes (1889 and 1892) to the dean of the faculty but this is all. Explanation for this situation may lie in the fact that considerable controversy arose respecting the administration of the school during this period, as explained in Chapter 7.
7 *Dominion Dental Journal*, October 1890
8 Throughout the text of this book, the name used for a dental organization is the one current at the time referred to. Several organizations altered their names from time to time, often for short periods. Ontario Dental Association was the name originally adopted in 1867, but the proceedings of the meeting held in July 1868 are entitled those of the Dental Association of Ontario. By 1869 the title Ontario Dental Society was in use, and this name prevailed, with one or two short interruptions, until 1920, when the organization was incorporated under the original name, Ontario Dental Association.
9 Text of an address by F.J. Conboy, *Dominion Dental Journal*, Vol 37, March 1925
10 Private correspondence with his grandson, now president of the company

CHAPTER 7   *Pages 81–99*

1 *Dominion Dental Journal*, Vol 2, No 3, July 1890
2 University of Trinity College Archives. The Archivist of Trinity states that there is no evidence that actual teaching of dentistry occurred there.
3 Bowmanville *Statesman*, July 1908
4 'J.M. Brimacombe – His Life,' *Dominion Dental Journal*, Vol 20, September 1908
5 Robert Tyre, *Saddlebag Surgeon: The Story of Dr Murrough O'Brien* (Toronto 1954)
6 *Dominion Dental Journal*, Vol 8, No 1, January 1896
7 Laval University at Montreal was a branch of Laval University at Quebec until 1920, when it became the University of Montreal.
8 The name of Josephine Wells appears on the Register of the Royal College of Dental Surgeons of Ontario, numbered 616.
9 Annie Grant Hill appears on the Register of the College of Dental Surgeons of the Province of Quebec, numbered 135.
10 In describing this machine at some length in its 18 June 1898 issue, *Scientific American* reported: 'It was rebuilt for winter use by Dr H.E. Casgrain of Quebec, Canada. It is an interesting development of the automobile vehicle and opens another field for those who are working on the important problem of automobile propulsion.'
11 Dental literature contains many references to the implantation of teeth by John Hunter. In a copy of his book, *A practical treatise on the diseases of the teeth* (London, 1778) appears a footnote: 'I may here just remark that the experiment is not generally attended with success. I succeeded but once out of a great

number of trials.' The author is indebted to Menzies Campbell of Glasgow for accuracy on this point.

12 Cataphoresis must not be confused with electrolytic medication (ionization) which came into use two decades later.

13 In part the statements respecting Frank Price are based upon private correspondence with his son, Dr Harold W. Price of Calgary.

14 On this point see Chapter 17.

15 In a letter to the secretary of the Provincial Board of Health, 10 February 1896, Adams stated that he had operated his dental hospital for 25 years.

16 *Dominion Dental Journal*, Vol 5, April 1893

17 *Dominion Dental Journal*, Vol 9, October 1897

18 Based on 1901 census figures

CHAPTER 8   *Pages 100–112*

1 From a 16-page booklet prepared and distributed by W.K. McNaught, proposing erection of a suitable memorial to Beers in the city of Montreal. Copies exist in several archives and libraries. McNaught was one of Toronto's leading businessmen of the period.

2 From 1896 to 1906 inclusive, Bishop's conferred 86 dental degrees, of which 26 were granted in 1896 to dentists who had already qualified with the Quebec Board. See D.C. Masters, *Bishop's University: The First Hundred Years* (Toronto, 1950)

3 Original documents in the library of McGill University

4 *Dominion Dental Journal*, Vol 14, No 3, March 1902

5 D.H. Baird's son, Kenneth Martin Baird, was Director-General Dental Services of the Royal Canadian Dental Corps, 1958–66.

6 *Dominion Dental Journal*, Vol 16, No 10, October 1904

7 This is one of the peculiarities found in the records. Juvet's name does not appear among the successful candidates at the first examination of the Dominion Dental Council. Seven candidates took the first examination, of whom four were successful: J.W. Coram, J.W. Clay, W.R. Glover, and E.C. Jones.

8 *Dominion Dental Journal*, Vol 12, No 1, January 1900

9 *Dominion Dental Journal*, Vol 16, No 3, March 1904

CHAPTER 9   *Pages 113–135*

1 *Dominion Dental Journal*, Vol 17, No 6, June 1905

2 Among recent articles about Parker are 'The Great Tycoon' (*True*, June 1956) and 'Painless Parker' (*Maclean's*, 15 December 1949). All through his career he gained a great deal of newspaper publicity in addition to his advertisements, which were often full-page in size.

3 *Dominion Dental Journal*, Vol 26, No 6, June 1914

4 *Le Bulletin des Recherches Historiques*, Vol 36, No 9, September 1930

5 Archives of Canadian Dental Association

6 The spelling in official documents during this era is 'North-West' and in other records it tends to be 'Northwest'.

7 Copy of the register is in the CDA archives.

8 Address delivered previous to the visit of William Hunter, *Dominion Dental Journal*, Vol 22, No 6, June 1910

9 *The Lancet*, 14 January 1911

10 Arthur W. Lufkin, *History of Dentistry* (Philadelphia, 1948)
11 For the most part this information was secured by personal interview with Dr Lindsay, just previous to his death in 1968.
12 The number of practising dentists in Canada who did not possess a university degree continued to diminish very rapidly. By the 1940s it became difficult to find, even among older practitioners, a dentist who did not hold a university degree.
13 The establishment of dental laboratories continued to be strongly opposed by some dentists, as the following item from the minutes of the 1910 annual meeting of the Quebec licentiates indicates: 'The matter of the King Dental Laboratory being brought up, Dr Masson complained of the harm that such laboratories were doing to young graduates. Drs Nolin, Mallet and Dubeau took part in the discussion and finally the matter was left with the Board.'
14 An editorial in the *Dominion Dental Journal*, Vol 17, No 9, September 1905, stated: 'It is a fact, and has been for years, that there are more Canadians obtaining their dental education in the United States than there are in Canada.'
15 *Dominion Dental Journal*, Vol 18, No 10, October 1906

CHAPTER 10   *Pages 136–149*

1 In 1968, a Royal Commission into Civil Rights, which had been appointed by the Ontario Government, reported at considerable length on the whole matter of self-government by the professions. Many matters respecting legal procedures in the conduct of proceedings by self-governing boards and councils were discussed with recommendations for improvement. Perhaps the most important recommended change was that lay members be appointed 'to each of the self-governing bodies of the self-governing professions and occupations,' in order to give protection to the public. However, the report emphasized that 'the educational training of members of the professions extends over many years and puts members of a profession in the best position to judge.'
2 For others so honoured, see Appendix H.
3 *Dominion Dental Journal*, Vol 26, No 5, May 1914
4 Personal communication with the author
5 Mr Gerald V. Carveth of Grande Prairie, in a personal communication
6 This was recognition by a public authority. Voluntary efforts by the Halifax Visiting Dispensary and J.G. Adams have been described in earlier chapters.
7 *Dominion Dental Journal*, Vol 23, No 10, October 1911
8 A good description is to be found in *The Britannica Year Book 1913*.

CHAPTER 11   *Pages 150–164*

1 Eventually, small payment was offered to these volunteer dentists, calculated at a rate of $3 per visit. A copy of a letter has survived, signed by twenty-five dentists who had served in this capacity, recording their appreciation for the money and returning the cheque in support of the military dental clinic.
2 Thornton was in his senior year at time of enlistment and his name appears in the 1917 class of McGill dental graduates. Ranks were allotted without complete regard to regulations in these first overseas units.
3 See *No 3 Canadian General Hospital in France* (published by McGill University in 1916) and R.C. Fetherstonaugh, *No 3 Canadian General Hospital (McGill) 1914–1919* (Montreal, 1928)

4 H.M. Jackson, *The Story of the Royal Canadian Dental Corps*. Several personal accounts of war experiences have appeared in dental literature. One of the best, 'Personal Reminiscences of a Field Ambulance Dental Officer,' by R.J. Godfrey, was published in the *Journal of the Ontario Dental Association*, Vol 42, No 8, August 1965.

5 'Canada Leads the Way,' reprinted from the *Canadian Gazette* (London), *Dominion Dental Journal*, Vol 30, No 4, April 1918

6 *Dominion Dental Journal*, Vol 32, No 9, September 1920

7 Considering that the x-ray was just beginning to come into general use in the dental office, the following extract from one of Hemingway's articles (*Toronto Star Weekly*, 10 April 1920) is notable: 'The x-ray is not infallible, according to dentists. Too many dentists accept the x-ray picture as final and order the tooth pulled. The x-ray should only be one step in the diagnosis. It may show almost anything, depending upon the angle from which it is taken and the skill of the dentist who is reading it.'

8 The government indicated that it would make the grant before the students were accepted, but an anxious period of delay occurred before the grant received formal government approval.

9 The basic reason for discontinuing the course then was that the University of Toronto raised the admission requirements in accord with those of all its other courses, and this action drastically reduced the number of applicants.

10 *Dominion Dental Journal*, Vol 35, No 1, January 1923

CHAPTER 12   *Pages 165–174*

1 *Dental Education in the United States and Canada*, Carnegie Foundation for the Advancement of Teaching, Bulletin No 19, 1926

2 *Proceedings of the Dental Centenary Celebrations (1840–1940)* (Baltimore, 1940)

3 *Dominion Dental Journal*, Vol 32, No 11, November 1920

4 Original copies of these circulars exist in the archives of the Canadian Dental Association.

5 *A Course of Study in Dentistry: Report of the Curriculum Survey Committee* (American Association of Dental Schools, 1935)

6 Today's debate centres on the position of the dentist in hospitals, health service plans, group practice, and similar matters.

7 Dentists in this era were faced with patients for whom the diagnosis was already made. Great tact and diplomacy were required in dealing with the situation, especially when the dentist knew that the diagnosis was incorrect.

8 *Dominion Dental Journal*, Vol 37, No 1, January 1925

9 *Dominion Dental Journal*, Vol 36, Nos 10 and 11, October and November 1924

CHAPTER 13   *Pages 175–185*

1 The records of the Canadian Dental Hygiene Council are deposited in the Archives of the Canadian Dental Association.

2 *Dominion Dental Journal*, Vol. 39, No 7, July 1927

3 See Appendix E, Establishment of Departments of Health in Canada.

4 The program of a combined meeting of the Dental Association of the Province of Nova Scotia and the New Brunswick Dental Society held at Amherst, NS, in

August 1900 contains the following item: 'Combination Gold and Amalgam Contour Fillings Using a Matrix by H.E. Bulyea.'

5 R.A. McEwen, at present a member of the teaching staff of the School of Dentistry, Emory University, Atlanta, Georgia, in a private communication

6 *Dominion Dental Journal,* Vol 39, No 5, May 1927. See Appendix I for PH D degrees earned in dentistry at Canadian universities.

7 'Résumé de l'évolution de la chirurgie-dentaire au Canada,' *Journal de l'Association Dentaire Canadienne,* October 1943

8 *Proceedings of the Royal College of Dental Surgeons of Ontario,* 1929–30

9 A transcript of this meeting is in the Archives of the Canadian Dental Association.

CHAPTER 14 *Pages 186–196*

1 Sylvister Moyer, 'The Practice of Dentistry in the Drought Area of the West,' *Journal of the Canadian Dental Association,* Vol 1, No 3, March 1935. The widow of a blacksmith requested that he accept the whole blacksmithing outfit in payment for a complete set of dentures. On this exchange the dentist did very well, but at a much later date.

2 Private interview with R.S. Langstroth of Fredericton.

3 *Journal of the Canadian Dental Association,* Vol 1, No 3, March 1935

4 *Dominion Dental Journal,* Vol 42, No 7, July 1930

5 *British Dental Journal,* Vol 53, No 7, 1 October 1932

6 The first is from the *Journal of the Ontario Dental Association,* Vol 7, No 8, August 1932; the second from the *Dominion Dental Journal,* Vol 46, No 1, January 1934

7 See Appendix G, Dental Journalism in Canada.

8 *Journal of the Ontario Dental Association,* Vol 7, No 9, September 1932

CHAPTER 15 *Pages 197–206*

1 *Study of the Distribution of Medical Care and Public Health in Canada (1939),* published by the National Committee for Mental Hygiene (Canada)

2 Canadian Dental Association, 'A Submission to the Royal Commission on Dominion-Provincial Relations,' 1938

3 *Report of the Royal Commission on Dominion-Provincial Relations* (the Rowell-Sirois Report) (Ottawa, 1940)

4 H.M. Jackson, *The Story of the Royal Canadian Dental Corps*

CHAPTER 16 *Pages 207–218*

1 Hugh H. Wolfenden, *A Memorandum for the Dental Profession on the Subject of National Health and Health Insurance* (December 1949); *Principles of a Dental Health Plan* (Royal College of Dental Surgeons of Ontario, February 1942); Don W. Gullett, *An Outline of Health Insurance Referring to Dentistry in Particular* (May 1942)

2 This presentation, together with others, was published by the Canadian Dental Association in *The Dental Profession in Canada and Health Insurance* (1944) and distributed to Canadian dentists.

3 The chairman of the government advisory committee had specifically stated that only two representatives of the profession should appear before the committee.
4 L.C. March, *Report on Social Security for Canada* (1943)
5 *Health Insurance*, Report of the Advisory Committee on Health Insurance to the House of Commons Special Committee on Social Security (Ottawa, 1943)
6 Proceedings of the Special Committee on Social Security of the House of Commons, May 1943
7 *Proceedings of the Canadian Dental Association*, 1943. This statement gave the representatives more concern than any other at the meeting.
8 *Journal of the Canadian Dental Association*, Vol 10, No 1, January 1944
9 J.W. Pickersgill and D. F. Forster, *The Mackenzie King Record*, Vol II (Toronto, 1968)
10 Canadian Medical Procurement and Assignment Board, *Report of the National Health Survey*
11 *Proceedings of the Royal College of Dental Surgeons of Ontario*, 1944

CHAPTER 17   *Pages 219–235*

1 The 1917 minutes of the Eastern Ontario Dental Association record the following motion: 'That in the establishment of the Federal Department of Health this Association feels that the importance of the profession of dentistry demands that it shall be fully recognized by and adequately represented in this department.' Subsequently other dental organizations took similar action, but this is the first recorded statement by the profession that dentistry should be a part of the proposed department.
2 See Chapter 7.
3 *Dominion Dental Journal*, Vol 21, No 1, January 1909
4 House of Commons Debates, May 1948
5 In 1946, Diplomas in Dental Public Health (DDPH) were awarded by the University of Toronto to H.K. Brown, S.L. Honey, F.A. Kohli, and H.R. McLaren. These were the first Canadian dentists to qualify.
6 These 17 dentists were graduates of the following dental schools: Dalhousie University, 6; Royal College of Dental Surgeons, 2; St Louis University, 2; McGill University, University of Toronto, Pennsylvania College of Dental Surgery, Georgetown University, University of Heidelberg, University of Dublin, Temple University, 1 each.

CHAPTER 18   *Pages 236–249*

1 At the 1917 General Assembly of the Licentiates of the Province of Quebec, a motion was presented instructing the Dental Board to establish a school for dental nurses. No action followed. The discussion which occurred at the time indicates that behind the motion was the valuable service of dental sergeants (assistants) in the Dental Corps during the first world war.
2 Mary A. Brett of Regina became the first registered dental hygienist in Canada in May 1950. She graduated from the School of Dental Hygiene of the University of Minnesota in 1948. Her father, A.J. Brett, was secretary of the Dominion Dental Council for many years.
3 *Transactions of the Canadian Dental Association*, 1952
4 *Journal of the Canadian Dental Association*, Vol 18, No 1, January 1952

Notes

1 See Appendix J, Canadian Dental Schools.
2 Harvard University established the first dental school under university discipline in the United States in 1867, and awarded the degree of Doctor of Dental Medicine to graduates. As of 1969, out of 52 dental schools in the United States, the graduates of 10 schools receive the DMD degree. Graduates of the other U.S. schools receive the Doctor of Dental Surgery (DDS) degree.
3 *Report of the Royal Commission on Health Services* (Ottawa, 1964)
4 See Appendix F, Dentists in the Parliament of Canada.
5 The number of women students in Canadian medical schools has risen notably in recent years. In 1968, more than 12 per cent of medical students were women; in 1964, it was reported that 7.6 per cent of active physicians in Canada were women. In comparison, the percentage of dental students who were women was 4.7 in 1968. The highest percentage of active women dentists was 2.3, in 1967.
6 Among many others, John Downer of Toronto during the 1920s invented the electrical device for heating hot water in general use in homes today, and A.H. Goodwin of Edmonton invented several devices for the use of natural gas early in this century. The inventions of H.E. Casgrain and William Green have been referred to in the text.
7 He is the only Canadian dentist appearing as an author in the *Oxford Companion to Canadian History and Literature*.

Appendices

A Dentists of 1858
B Petition to the Ontario Legislature, 1868
C The World's First Dental Act: Ontario, 1868
D Canadian Dental Organizations, 1905
E Establishment of Departments of Health in Canada
F Dentists in the Parliament of Canada
G Dental Journalism in Canada
H Honorary Degrees Conferred on Canadian Dentists
I Degrees of Doctor of Philosophy Earned by Graduates of Canadian Dental Schools
J Canadian Dental Schools
K Recommendations by the Canadian Dental Association to the Royal Commission on Health Services, 1962

A   Dentists listed in directories for the year 1858
     (Population figures given in parentheses)

NOVA SCOTIA

Halifax (25,126)   M.F. Agnew
                          S. Foss
                          N.A. Glover
                          McAllister & Paine
                          L.E. VanBuskirk

NEW BRUNSWICK

Saint John (27,300)   C.K. Fiske
                          T.A.D. Forester
                          J.C. Hathaway
Fredericton   Mr Archer
                          Hiram Dow
Woodstock   W.A. Balloch

CANADA EAST

Quebec (51,000)   Pierre Baillargeon
                          John McKee
                          H.D. Ross
Montreal (75,000)   C.M. Dickinson
                          Charles Brewster
                          George VanBuskirk
                          H.M. Bowker
                          Aldis Bernard
Sherbrooke (3,000)   None listed
Three Rivers (7,000)   None listed
Waterloo (1,500)   None listed

CANADA WEST

Belleville (7,000)   G.V.N. Relyea
Brantford (8,000)   J.N. Acret
                          John P. Sutton
Brockville (5,000)   T.W. Smythe
Cobourg (7,000)   F.G. Callander
Galt (3,000)   R. Reid
Guelph (4,500)   Henry S.M. Swift

Hamilton (29,000)	C.S. Chittenden
	George S. Smith
	Myles B. Stennett
	John Reid
Kingston (13,000)	B.W. Day
London (16,000)	D.G. French
	A.C. Stone
	Darius Perrin
Ottawa (10,000)	F.D. Laughlin
Newmarket (1,000)	R. Moore
Perth (2,500)	G.W. Ebertson
Picton (2,000)	W.H. Gilbert
Port Hope (5,000)	S.B. Chandler
Prescott (4,000)	Edwin Church
St Catharines (6,500)	J. Harrison
	Francis Smith
St Mary's (2,500)	John McLean
Toronto (50,000)	W.C. Adams
	George L. Elliott
	John W. Elliott
	Mortimer French
	J.B. Jones
Whitby (3,500)	Justice S. Jones
Zimmerman (60)	Johnson Zimmerman

The source of the above information is the *Canada Directory* (Canada East and Canada West), published in 1858, and directories for Nova Scotia and New Brunswick published in the same year. These directories list by muncipalities each resident with his occupation. The directories are restricted however to more or less permanent residents: they would not take into account itinerant dentists nor the tendency of other practitioners to move often from place to place in search of a better location. Names other than those above are to be found in the dental literature. For example, L. Clements stated, some thirty years later, that he had established practice at Kingston in September 1857, but probably he was not considered a resident when the directory was compiled. The above information gives some relative idea only of 'established' practice at that time.

B   Petition to the Ontario Legislature

An exact copy of the petition presented to the Ontario Legislature by the
Ontario Dental Association, 23 January 1868. The original reposes in the
Ontario Archives, Toronto.

PETITION.

*To the Honorable the Legislative Assembly of the Province of Ontario, in Parliament
assembled,*

YOUR PETITIONERS RESPECTFULLY REPRESENT,

Whereas, it is expedient for the protection of the public, that there should, by enactment, be established a certain standard of qualification, required of each person practising the profession or calling of Dentistry in this Province,

We therefore pray, that an Act be passed requiring that persons so practising shall be examined by a competent Board, as to their qualifications to practice the said profession or calling.

NAME.	OCCUPATION.	RESIDENCE.

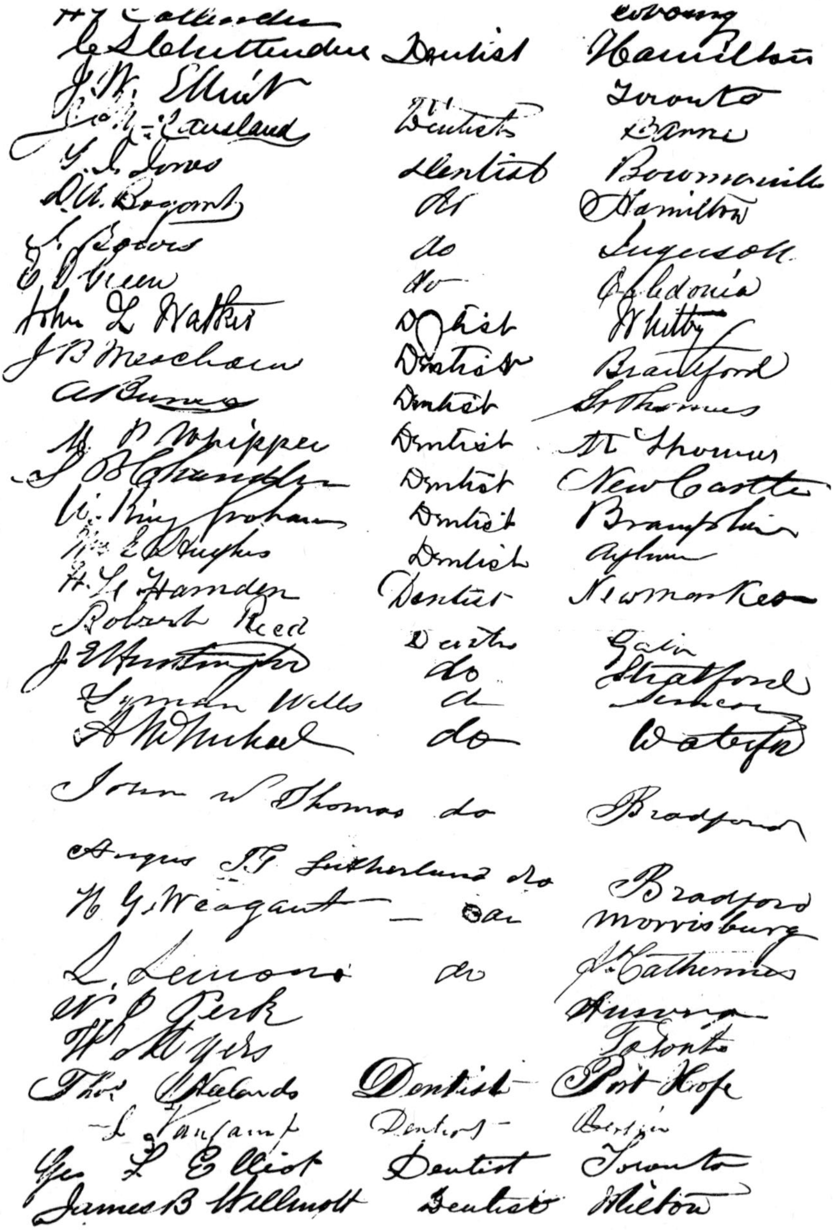

H J Callender		Cobourg
C S Chittenden	Dentist	Hamilton
J. W. Elliot		Toronto
[illegible] McCausland	Dentists	Barrie
[illegible] Jones	Dentist	Bowmanville
D. A. Bogart	do	Hamilton
[illegible] Eddows	do	Ingersoll
[illegible] Green	do	Caledonia
John L Walker	Dentist	Whitby
J B Meacham	Dentist	Brantford
A Burns	Dentist	St Thomas
H P Whipper	Dentist	St Thomas
S B Chandler	Dentist	New Castle
[illegible] King Graham	Dentist	Brampton
[illegible] E Hughes	Dentist	Aylmer
H L Hamden	Dentist	Newmarket
Robert Reed	Dentist	Galt
J E Huntington	do	Stratford
Lyman Wells	do	Simcoe
A McMichael	do	Waterloo
John W Thomas	do	Bradford
Angus J T Sutherland	do	Bradford
H G Weagant	do	Morrisburg
L Lemon	do	St Catharines
W [illegible] Peck		Aurora
W [illegible] Myers		Toronto
Thos Rowlands	Dentist	Port Hope
L Vangamp	Dentist	Berlin
Geo L Elliot	Dentist	Toronto
James B Willmott	Dentist	Milton

A. C. Stone, M.D.   Dentist   London
J. M. Brimacombe   Dentist   Bowmanville
Wm. H. Porter   Dentist   Holland Landing
J. Zimmer   Dentist   Zimmerm
54
R. D. LaGorÜe   Dentist   Brockville
Andrew May.   Dentist   St. Catharines
David Rutleus   Dentist   Peterboro

Geo. W. Hale   Dentist   Toronto
J. M. Wells   Dentist   Aurora
A. S. Rupert   Dentist   St. Mary's
60
J. R. Irish   Dentist

John Rolph, LL.D. M.D.
M R C S Eng.
Professor Med. Vic. Coll.
A. C. Stone M.D.   Dentist   London
Jos Adams   do   do
                          do   do
H. H. Nelles DDS   do   do
                                      do
David Perrin S.D.
C. Hampbell, M.D.   do

Leggs   Physician & Surgeon   Ottawa City
Charles A. Mondelet   Surgeon Dentist   Ottawa City
Jno Legg   do   do   Ottawa City
Charles Bonyman A.M. M.D.   Yorkville
Member of Municipal Council
Ont.   Physician

E. P. Barrick M.D. L R C P S
M R C S Eng.   Toronto

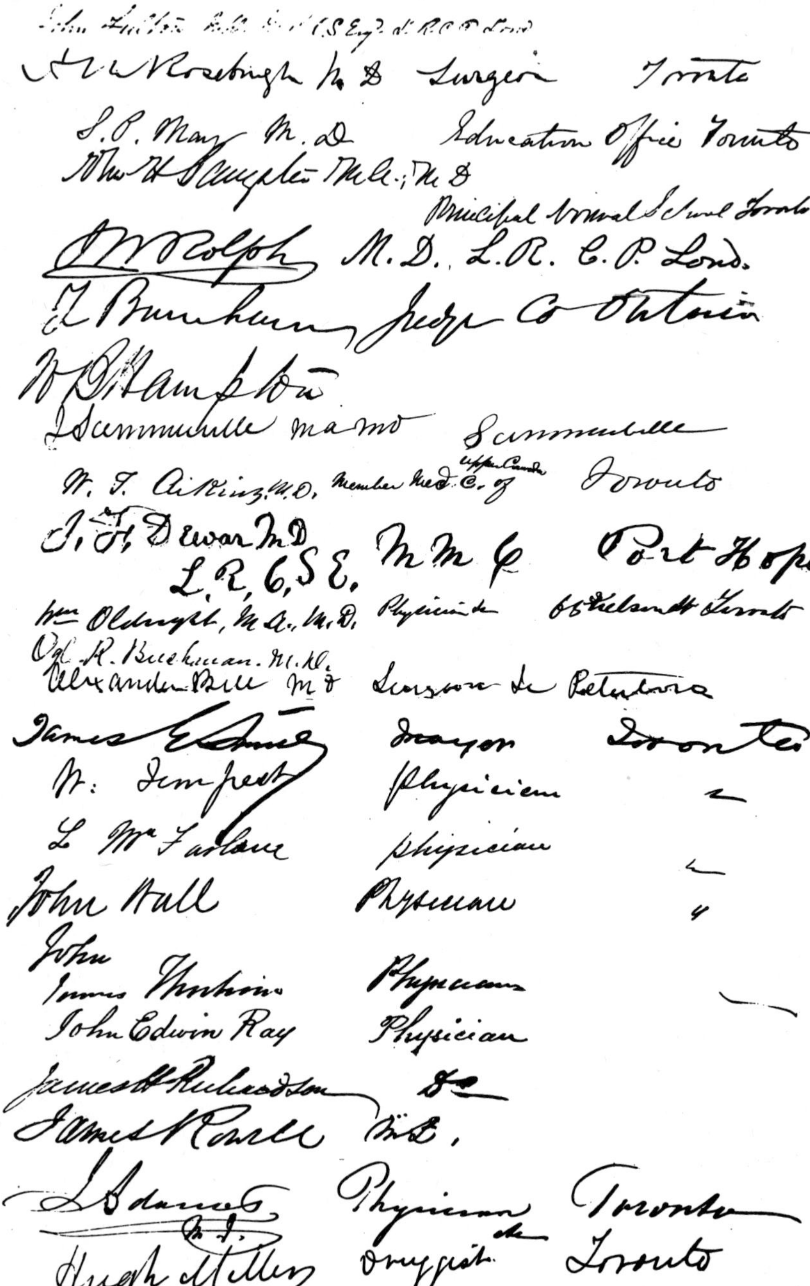
John Fulton M.D. M.R.C.S. Eng. & L.R.C.P. Lond

J. W. Rosebrugh M.D. Surgeon Toronto

S. P. May M.D. Education Office Toronto

Jno H Sangster M.A.; M.D. Principal Normal School Toronto

J. W. Rolph M.D. L.R.C.P. Lond.

Z. Burnham Judge Co Ontario

W. D. Hampton

J. Sommerville M.A. M.D. Sommerville

W. T. Aikins M.D. Member Med. C. of Upper Canada Toronto

J. F. Dewar M.D. L.R.C.S.E. M.M.C. Port Hope

Wm Oldright, M.A., M.D. Physician &c 66 Nelson St Toronto

Ogd. R. Buchanan M.D.

Alexander Bell M.D. Surgeon &c Peterboro

James E. Smith Mayor Toronto

W. Tempest Physician "

L. McFarlane Physician "

John Hall Physician "

John James Watson Physicians "

John Edwin Ray Physician

James H Richardson do

James Rowell M.D.

L. Adams M.D. Physician Toronto

Hugh Miller Druggist &c Toronto

C   The world's first dental Act, Ontario, 1868

A copy of the Act, reproduced by courtesy of the Ontario Archives, Toronto

CAP. XXXVII.

An Act respecting Dentistry.

[Assented to 4th March, 1868.]

Preamble.

WHEREAS the profession of Dentistry is extensively practised in the Province of Ontario, and whereas it is expedient for the protection of the public, that there should by enactment be established a certain standard of qualification required of each practitioner of the said profession, and that certain privileges and protection should be afforded to such practitioners: Therefore Her Majesty, by and with the advice and consent of the Legislative Assembly of Ontario, enacts as follows:

Incorporation by name.

1. The persons named in Section two of this Act shall be incorporated and known as the "Royal College of Dental Surgeons of Ontario."

2.

2. Until other persons be elected as hereinafter Provisional Board of Trustees and Examiners. provided, Barnabas W. Day, of the City of Kingston, M. D.; Curtis Strong Chittenden, of the City of Hamilton; Henry Tunstall Wood, of the Town of Picton; John O'Donnell, of the Town of Peterborough; Joseph Stuart Scott, of the City of Toronto, M. D.; Franklin Goodrich Callender, of the Town of Cobourg; George Van Nest Relyea, of the Town of Belleville; Antoine Denmark Lalonde, of the Town of Brockville; Charles Kahn, of the Town of Stratford, and James Bogart Meacham, of the Town of Brantford, and George L. Elliot of the City of Toronto, and John Leggo of the City of Ottawa, shall be trustees and a Board Quorum. of Examiners, of whom five shall be a quorum, to examine and grant certificates of license to practice Dental Surgery in this Province.

3. The Board of Directors to be elected, as hereinafter men- Directors to hold office for two years. tioned, shall consist of twelve members, who shall hold office for two years; any member may at any time resign by letter directed to the Secretary, and in the event of such resignation, or a vacancy occurring by death or otherwise, the remaining members of the Board shall elect some fit and proper person Vacancies. from among the licentiates to supply such vacancy.

4. The first election shall take place on the first Tuesday in First Election. June, one thousand eight hundred and sixty-eight, at such place, in the city of Toronto, as shall be fixed by by-law of the Provisional Board, and the Secretary of such Board shall act as Returning Officer at said election, and the persons qualified to vote at such election shall be the Licentiates of said Provisional Board, admitted without examination, as provided by section twelve of this Act, at least one month before said election, and the said Provisional Board shall issue such certificates to such persons upon their compliance with the requisites of said section, and it shall be the duty of the Secretary to publish in the *Ontario Gazette*, for two weeks immediately after said election, the names of the persons who have been elected members of the Board.

5. The said newly elected Board, as well as all Boards to be First meeting of Board. hereafter elected, shall hold their first meeting on the third Tuesday in July, next after the said elections in the city of Toronto, at such place as may be fixed by the Board.

6. Every subsequent election shall be held on the first Subsequent elections. Tuesday in June, in every second year, after the said first election, and the persons qualified at the said election shall be those Licentiates who have obtained their certificates as provided for in the twelfth section of this Act.

7. The said Board shall, at their first meeting after their elec- Appointment of a President and other officers. tion, elect from among themselves a President, Treasurer, Secretary and Registrar, and such other officers as may be necessary to
the

the working of this Act and the rules and regulations of said Board; and the said Board shall, from time to time, in the event of the President being absent, from any cause whatever, elect, from among their number, a person to preside at their meetings, who shall have the same powers, and exercise the same functions, as the President.

Remuneration.

8. There shall be allowed and paid to each of the members of said Board such fees for attendances (in no case to exceed five dollars per day and such reasonable travelling expenses) as shall from time to time be allowed by said Board.

Funds payable to the Treasurer.

9. All moneys forming part of the funds of said Board shall be paid to the Treasurer, and shall be applied to the carrying of this Act into execution.

Curriculum of Studies to be fixed by the Board.

Students to be articled.

Examination and fees payable before License to practice.

10. The Board shall have power and authority to establish and conduct a Dental College in Toronto, to appoint Professors, to fix and determine from time to time a curriculum of studies to be pursued by students, and to fix and determine the period for which every student shall be articled and employed under some duly licensed practitioner, and the examination necessary to be passed before said Board, and the fees to be paid into the hands of the Treasurer of said Board, before receiving a certificate of license to practise the profession of dentistry.

Sittings of the Board for examination of Students, &c.

11. The said Board may hold two sittings in every year for the purpose of examining students, granting certificates of license, and doing such other business as may properly come before them, such sittings to commence on the third Tuesday in July and January, in each and every year, which may be continued by adjournment from day to day, until the business before the said Board be finished, but no session shall exceed one week, said sittings to be held in the City of Toronto.

Who entitled to certificates.

12. All persons being British subjects by birth or naturalization, who have not been constantly engaged for five years in established office practice next preceding the passing of this act in the practice of the profession of dentistry, shall be entitled to a certificate of Licentiate of Dental Surgery, upon their furnishing to the said Board satisfactory proof of their having been so engaged, and upon passing the required examination, and upon payment of such fees as may be authorized and fixed by the said Board, for the payment of which the Treasurer's receipt shall be sufficient evidence, and all persons being British subjects, by birth or naturalization, who have been constantly engaged for five years and upwards in established office practice, next preceding the passing of this Act, in the practice of the profession of dentistry, shall, upon such proof as aforesaid, and upon the payment of the fees as aforesaid, be entitled to such certificate without passing any examination.

13.

13. The said Board shall at its first meeting, and from time to time thereafter, make such rules, regulations and by-laws as may be necessary for the proper and better guidance, government and regulation of said Board and College, and said profession of Dentistry, as to fees and otherwise, and the carrying out of this Act; which said rules, regulations and by-laws, shall be published for two consecutive weeks in the Ontario *Gazette*; any or all of such rules, regulations and by-laws shall be liable to be cancelled and annulled by an order of the Lieutenant-Governor of this Province. *The Board to make Rules, Regulations and By-laws. Publication in the Ontario Gazette.*

14. Every person desirous of being examined by the said Board, touching his qualifications for the practice of the profession of dentistry, shall at least one month before the sittings of said Board, pay into the hands of the Treasurer the required fees, and inclose and deliver to the Secretary the Treasurer's receipt for the same, together with satisfactory evidences of his apprenticeship, integrity and good morals; and it shall be the duty of the Board to hold a sitting for the purpose hereinbefore mentioned, on the third Tuesdays of January and July, whichever shall first happen, next ensuing the said payment and delivery. *Fees payable before examination.*

15. If the Board be satisfied by the examination that the person is duly qualified to practise the profession of Dentistry, and be further satisfied that he is a person of integrity and good moral character, they shall grant him a certificate of license and the title of Licentiate of Dental Surgery, which certificate and title shall entitle him to all the rights and privileges of this Act until such time as the Board shall be satisfied that he has been guilty of acts, detrimental to the interests of the profession, when he shall forfeit his certificate, and it shall be cancelled; such forfeiture may, however, be waived, and the said certificate of License and all rights and privileges thereunder, fully revived by said Board, in such manner and upon such terms and conditions as to said Board may seem expedient. *Certificate of License. Designation of Title. Forfeiture, when.*

16. Every certificate of license shall be sealed with the Corporation Seal and signed by the President and Secretary of said Board; and the production of such certificate of license shall be *prima facie* evidence in all courts of law and upon all proceedings of whatever kind, of its execution and contents. *Certificate to be under the Corporate seal.*

17. The Secretary of the said Board shall, on or before the fifteenth day of January in each and every year, inclose to the Provincial Secretary a certified list of the names of all persons to whom certificates of license have been granted during the then next preceding year. *Certified lists of Licenses granted to be enclosed to the Provincial Secretary annually.*

18. If any person, after the period of twelve months after the passing of this Act, not holding a valid and unforfeited certificate of license, practises the said profession of Dentistry for hire, gain or hope of reward, or wilfully and falsely pretends *Persons practising without License to be guilty of misdemeanor.*

to

to hold a certificate of license under this Act, or takes or uses any name, title, addition or description implying that he is duly authorized to practise the said profession of Dentistry, or shall falsely use any title representing that he is a graduate of any Dental College either in Great Britain or other countries he shall be liable to a summary conviction, before any two or more Justices of the Peace, for every such offence, and shall, on such conviction, be liable to a fine not exceeding twenty dollars, which said penalty, in default of payment, shall be enforced by distress and sale of the offender's goods and chattels; and it is further provided that no such person shall recover in any Court of Law for any work done or materials provided by him in the ordinary and customary work of a Dentist.

Penalty not exceeding $20, upon summary conviction before any Justice.

In default of payment, imprisonment.

Inability to recover for work done.

This Act not to interfere with Physicians or Surgeons.

19. Nothing in this Act shall interfere with the privileges conferred upon Physicians and Surgeons by the various acts relating to the practice of Medicine and Surgery in this Province.

D   Canadian dental organizations, 1905

A page from the *Dominion Dental Journal*, April 1905

Directory of Official and Voluntary Dental Associations and Societies of Canada

OFFICIAL

NOVA SCOTIA DENTAL BOARD.

President—Hibbart Woodbury, D.D.S., Halifax, N.S.
Secretary—Geo. K. Thomson, D.D.S., Halifax, N.S.

PRINCE EDWARD ISLAND.

President—Dr. J. E. McDonald, Summerside, P.E.I.
Secretary—Dr. J. H. Ayers, Charlottetown, P.E.I.

NEW BRUNSWICK DENTAL SOCIETY.

President—J. W. Moore, D.D.S., St. John, N.B.
Secretary—Frank A. Godsoe, D.D.S., St. John, N.B.

QUEBEC DENTAL BOARD OF EXAMINERS.

President—G. E. Hyndman, D.D.S., Sherbrooke Que.

Secretary—Eudore Dubeau, D.D.S., 396 St. Denis
   Street, Montreal, Que.

BOARD OF THE ROYAL COLLEGE OF DENTAL SURGEONS OF ONTARIO.

President—H. R. Abbott, D.D.S., London, Ont.
Secretary—J. B. Willmott, D.D.S., 96 College Street, Toronto, Ont.

MANITOBA DENTAL ASSOCIATION.

President—G. J. Clint, D.D.S., Winnipeg, Man.
Secretary—G. F. Bush, D.D.S., Winnipeg, Man.

NORTH-WEST TERRITORIES DENTAL ASSOCIATION.

President—R. C. McLure, D.D.S., Lethbridge, Assa.
Secretary—P. F. Size, D.D.S., Moosejaw, Assa.

BRITISH COLUMBIA DENTAL ASSOCIATION.

President—T. J. Jones, D.D.S., Victoria, B.C.
Secretary—Richard Nash, D.D.S., Victoria, B.C.

YUKON DENTAL BOARD.

President—A. J. Gillis, M.D., D.D.S., Dawson, Y.T.
Secretary—C. H. Wells, L.D.S., Dawson, Y.T.

VOLUNTARY

CANADIAN DENTAL ASSOCIATION.

President—Eudore Dubeau, Montreal.
Secretary—Dr. C. F. Morison, 14 Phillip Square, Montreal.

MARITIME DENTAL ASSOCIATION.

President— —. McArthur, D.D.S., Truro, N.S.
Secretary—G. K. Thompson, D.D.S., Halifax, N.S.

DENTAL SOCIETY OF WESTERN CANADA.

President—S. W. McInnis, D.D.S., Brandon, Man.
Secretary—C. P. Banning, D.D.S., McIntyre Building, Winnipeg, Man.

ONTARIO DENTAL SOCIETY.

President—A. W. Thornton, D.D.S., Chatham, Ont.
Secretary—Guy G. Hume, D.D.S., 228 Carlton Street, Toronto, Ont.

LA SOCIETE D'ODONTOLOGIC CANADIENNE FRANCAISE

President—Joseph Nolin, Montreal.
Secretary—Eudore Dubeau, 396 St. Denis Street, Montreal.

EASTERN ONTARIO DENTAL SOCIETY.

President—W. J. Gunn, D.D.S., Cornwall, Ont.
Secretary—W. B. Cavanagh, D.D.S., Cornwall, Ont.

WESTERN ONTARIO DENTAL SOCIETY.

President—J. Mills, D.D.S., Brantford, Ont.
Secretary—C. E. Snell, D.D.S., Essex Centre, Ont.

BRANT COUNTY DENTAL SOCIETY.

President—John Mills.
Secretary—F. Britton.

LONDON DENTAL SOCIETY.

President—A. E. Santo, D.D.S., London, Ont.
Secretary—S. Campbell, D.D.S., London, Ont.

ELGIN COUNTY DENTAL SOCIETY.

President—G. T. Kennedy, St. Thomas, Ont.
Secretary—C. B. Taylor, D.D.S., St. Thomas, Ont.

TORONTO DENTAL SOCIETY.

President—Chas. E. Pearson, Toronto.
Secretary—C. Angus Kennedy, 738 Queen St. East, Toronto, Ont.

MONTREAL DENTAL CLUB.

President—G. W. Oliver, 2681 St. Catherine Street, Montreal.
Secretary—W. Watson, D.D.S., 48 Park Ave., Montreal.

The above is a correct list of the dental organizations of Canada, with Presidents and Secretaries, so far as they are known to the Journal.   It is the intention to keep a list of the officers of all Canadian societies in the Journal, so where there are omissions or errors please notify the Editor, who will make the correction, and so far as possible keep a corrected list, which will be of great value to the organizations.

E   Establishment of Departments of Health and Divisions of
     Dental Health

	Department	Dental Division
Federal Government	1919	1945
British Columbia	1946	1949
Alberta	1919	1959
Saskatchewan	1923	1948
Manitoba	1928	1946
Ontario	1923	1925
Quebec	1926	1943
New Brunswick	1918	1948
Nova Scotia	1930	1948
Prince Edward Island	1931	1950
Newfoundland	1950	1952

Departments of Health in provincial governments were preceded by Provincial
Boards of Health.

New Brunswick was the first province to establish a department of health and
Ontario was first to establish a dental division. The Rowell-Sirois Commission
Report contains the following statement: 'New Brunswick alone of the
provinces had established a permanent board of health in 1866.'

F   Dentists in the Parliament of Canada

SENATE

Baillargeon, Pierre	1874–91
Phillips, Orville Howard	1963–
Smith, Donald	1955–

HOUSE OF COMMONS	*Year(s) Elected*
Armstrong, Ernest Frederick	1925
Buchanan, William Murdock	1953
Cowan, Walter Davy	1917–30
Duguay, Joseph Leonard	1930
Fauteux, Gaspard	1942–45–49
(Speaker of House, 1945–9;	
Member of the Privy Council, 1949;	
Lieutenant-Governor of Quebec 1950–8)	
Haley, Allen	1896
Hall, William Samuel	1935
Larue, Perrault	1958
Leduc, Rodolphe	1936–40–54–58–62–63
Mang, Henry Philip	1953
McDougall, John Lorne	1949–53
McKay, Matthew	1921–35
Phillips, Orville Howard	1957–58–62
Pommer, William Albert	1953
Price, Otto Baird	1925–26–30
Richard, Charles	1958
Slogan, Joseph	1958–62
Smith, Donald	1949
Stewart, John Smith	1930

G Dental journalism in Canada

THE FAMILY DENTIST published by S.S. Blodgett, Brockville, Ontario, 1854–?.
A few issues only, number unknown

THE JOURNAL OF THE TIMES published quarterly by MacAllister & Paine at
Halifax, Nova Scotia. First issue dated September 1858; last issue May and
June 1860; seven issues in all
(The above two publications were individual efforts and more in the nature of
promotion for the respective practices than true journalism.)

CANADA JOURNAL OF DENTAL SCIENCE published monthly at Montreal, except
for one year at Hamilton. EDITOR W. George Beers. Really the pioneer dental
journal in Canada. First issue June 1868. Volumes 1, 2 and 3 complete. Four
widely separated issues in volume 4 appeared, the last being August 1879

DOMINION DENTAL JOURNAL published at Toronto, quarterly 1889–90,
bimonthly 1891–2, monthly 1893–1934 (Vol 1–46).
EDITORS
W. George Beers   1889–1900
Albert E. Webster   1901–1934
The Dominion Dental Journal absorbed the *Canada Journal of Dental Science*
(1889), and in turn was taken over by the *Journal of the Canadian Dental
Association* (1935)

ASH'S CANADIAN MONTHLY CIRCULAR published at Toronto 1910–19 (Vol 1–9).
Began as a monthly and ended as a quarterly (Ash's Canadian Quarterly)

DENTAL PRACTICE published monthly at Toronto 1906–13 (Vol 1–14, two
volumes a year).
EDITOR Robert J. Reade
Became merged with a medical journal

ORAL HEALTH published monthly at Toronto 1911 to the present.
EDITORS
Wallace Seccombe   1911–35
Thomas Cowling   1936–50
Wesley J. Dunn   1951–53
J.H. Johnson   1953–66
D.B. McAdam   1966–68
J.M. Kerr   1969–

REVUE DENTAIRE CANADIENNE published monthly at Montreal 1918–34 (Vol 1–17).
EDITOR Honoré Thibault
Absorbed by *Journal of Canadian Dental Association* (1935)

JOURNAL OF THE ONTARIO DENTAL ASSOCIATION published monthly at Toronto. Vol 1–6, No 5, 1926, under title of *The Booster*. Vol 6, No 6, 1931 to date under title of *The Journal of the Ontario Dental Association*.
EDITORS
F.J. Conboy   1926–42
E.A. Grant   1942–45
G.T. Mitton   1945 (November and December only)
S.L. Honey   1946–51
A.W. Lindsay   1952–67
J.H. Johnson   1967–69
C.F. Cappa   1970–

JOURNAL OF THE CANADIAN DENTAL ASSOCIATION published monthly at Toronto 1935 to the present. Absorbed *Dominion Dental Journal* and *Revue Dentaire Canadienne* (1935)
EDITORS
M.H. Garvin   1935–53 (including June issue)
W.J. Dunn   1953–58
E.R. Bilkey   1959–60
F.H. Compton   1960–
FRENCH EDITORS
Philippe Hamel   1935–36
Alcide Thibaudeau   1937–46
Gerard deMontigny   1946–64
Georges Pelletier   1965–68
M. Tenenbaum   1969–

ADDITIONAL PUBLICATIONS
The following are currently published:
Royal Canadian Dental Corps Quarterly (Vol 1, 1960), Ottawa.
B.C. Dental Bulletin (formerly B.C.D.A. News), College of Dental Surgeons of British Columbia, Vancouver.
A.D.A. News-Information, Alberta Dental Association, Edmonton.
College of Dental Surgeons of Saskatchewan Newsletter, Saskatoon.

The Bulletin, Manitoba Dental Association, Winnipeg.

Information, College of Dental Surgeons of the Province of Quebec, Montreal.

Le Journal dentaire du Quebec (Vol 1, 1963), L'Association dentaire de la Province de Québec, Montréal.

N.S.D.A. News, Nova Scotia Dental Association, Halifax.

Bulletin mensuel de la Société dentaire de Montréal, Montréal.

Mount Royal Dental Society News Letter, Montreal.

McGill Dental Review, McGill University Undergraduate Dental Society, annual from 1934, now biannual, Montreal.

University of Toronto Undergraduate Dental Journal (Vol 1, 1964), three issues per volume, Toronto. This journal replaced *Hya Yaka* (Vol 1, No 1, October 1903) issued monthly (ten issues per year) until 1929, when it became an annual.

University of Western Ontario Dental Students Society Journal (Vol 1, 1966–7). Annual. London, Ontario.

Dalhousie Dental Journal (Vol 1, 1960). Annual. Halifax.

H   Honorary degrees conferred on Canadian dentists

1914   J.B. Willmott   LLD, University of Toronto
1919   Frank Woodbury   LLD, Dalhousie University
1932   A.E. Webster   LLD, University of Toronto
1943   Frank M. Lott   DDS, Université de Montréal
1945   A.W. Lindsay   LLD, University of Toronto
1950   John Clay   LLD, University of Alberta
1953   W.W. Woodbury   LLD, Dalhousie University
1954   A.J. Coughlan   BSC, St Joseph's University
1957   J.S. Stewart   LLD, University of Alberta
       M.H. Garvin   LLD, University of Manitoba
1958   D.W. Gullett   DDS, Université de Montréal
       A.J. Coughlan   LLD, Dalhousie University
       Ernest Charron   LLD, Dalhousie University
       D.W. Gullett   LLD, Dalhousie University
1959   A.D.A. Mason   LLD, University of Toronto
1960   H.J. Merkeley   LLD, University of Manitoba
       J.S. Bagnall   LLD, Dalhousie University
       H.E. Bulyea   LLD, University of Manitoba
1961   H.K. Brown   LLD, University of Alberta
1962   J.B. Macdonald   LLD, University of Manitoba
1963   D.W. Gullett   DSC, Temple University
1967   J.B. Macdonald   DSC, University of British Columbia
1968   R.G. Ellis   LLD, University of Western Ontario
1969   George F. Clarke   LLD, University of New Brunswick

I   Degrees of Doctor of Philosophy earned by graduates of Canadian
    dental schools up to 1969

1920   Harold K. Box   University of Toronto (Pathology)
1940   F.M. Lott   University of Toronto (Military Dentistry)
1941   R.G. Agnew   University of Toronto (Oral Pathology)
1950   S.W.Leung   University of Rochester (Physiology)
1953   J.B. Macdonald   Columbia University (Microbiology)
1953   K.J. Paynter   Columbia University (Anatomy)
1958   John Findlay   Glasgow University (Endocrinology)
1958   I. Kleinberg   University of Durham (Biochemistry)
1959   Grant T. Phipps   Pennsylvania State University (Psychology)
1959   W. Stuart Hunter   University of Michigan (Anthropology)
1959   J.P. Lussier   University of California (Endocrinology)
1959   Oscar P. Sykora   University of Montreal (Slavic Languages)
1963   R.V. Blackmore   University of Rochester (Microbiology)
1964   M.C. Johnson   University of Rochester (Embryology)
1964   A.T. Storey   University of Michigan (Physiology)
1965   Trevor Harrop   University of Iowa (Anatomy)
1967   H.W. Kaufman   University of Manitoba (Oral Biology)
1967   N.S. Taichman   University of Toronto (Immunopathology)
1967   James Sanaham   University of Manitoba (Oral Biology)
1968   A. Ian Hamilton   University of London (Anatomy)
1969   J.E. Stakiw   University of Manitoba (Oral Biology)

J   Canadian dental schools

Royal College of Dental Surgeons (Established 1875)*
DEANS
J.B. Willmott   1875–1915
A.E. Webster   1915–23
Wallace Seccombe   1923–5
Became Faculty of University of Toronto in 1925

Faculty of Dentistry, University of Toronto
DEANS
Wallace Seccombe   1925–36
A.D.A. Mason   1936–47
R.G. Ellis   1947–69
Gordon Nikiforuk   1970–

The Dental College of the Province of Quebec (Established 1892)
DEAN
W. George Beers   1892–6
Became a part of University of Bishop's College in 1896

Faculty of Dentistry, University of Bishop's College
DEANS
W. George Beers   1896
J.H. Bourdon (acting)   1897
Stephen Globensky   1897–9
J.G. Globensky   1899–1900
W.J. Kerr   1900–1
W.J. Giles   1901–2
Peter Brown   1902–4
Became two schools in 1905: Department of Dentistry of the Faculty of
Medicine, McGill University; and École de chirurgie dentaire, Université Laval

École de chirurgie dentaire, Université Laval
DOYEN
Eudore Dubeau   1905–21
Became Faculty, Université de Montréal in 1921

*'Established' signifies the year when the first class of students was accepted by the
school

Appendices

Faculté de chirurgie dentaire, Université de Montréal
DOYENS
Eudore Dubeau   1921–44
Ernest Charron   1944–58
Paul Geoffrion   1959–64
Jean-Paul Lussier   1964–

Department of Dentistry, Faculty of Medicine, McGill University
HEADS
Peter Brown   1905–9
D.J. Berwick 1910–13
A.W. Thornton   1913–20
Became Faculty of McGill University in 1920

Faculty of Dentistry, McGill University
DEANS
A.W. Thornton   1920–7
A.L. Walsh   1927–48
D.P. Mowry   1948–55
James McCutcheon   1955–70
E.R. Ambrose   1970–

Maritime Dental College (Established 1908)
DEAN
Frank Woodbury   1908–12
Became Faculty of Dalhousie University in 1912

Faculty of Dentistry, Dalhousie University
DEANS
Frank Woodbury   1912–22
Frank W. Ryan   1922–4
George K. Thompson   1924–35
W.W. Woodbury   1935–47
J. Stanley Bagnall   1947–54
J.D. McLean   1954–

Department of Dentistry, Faculty of Medicine, University of Alberta
(Established 1918)
DIRECTOR
H.E. Bulyea   1918–42
Became Faculty of University of Alberta in 1942

Faculty of Dentistry, University of Alberta
DEANS
W. Scott Hamilton   1942–58
H.R. MacLean   1958–70
James McCutcheon   1970–

Faculty of Dentistry, University of Manitoba (Established 1958)
DEAN
J.W. Neilson   1957–

Faculty of Dentistry, University of British Columbia (Established 1964)
DEAN
S. Wah Leung   1962–

Faculty of Dentistry, University of Western Ontario (Established 1966)
DEAN
W.J. Dunn   1965–

College of Dentistry, University of Saskatchewan (Established 1968)
DEAN
K.J. Paynter   1967–

Section de chirurgie dentaire, Centre des Sciences de la Santé, Université Laval
DIRECTEUR
Gustave Ratté   1968–

NOTES:
1   The Royal College of Dental Surgeons of Ontario operated a school for a few months during the winter of 1869–70, at Toronto, and graduated two students.
2   The Canada College of Dentistry (1869–71) was operated at Toronto by George L. Elliott, LDS. Records exist of seven graduates from this school and there may have been more. This was the only attempt in Canada to operate a private school.
3   Faculty of Dentistry, University of Trinity College, Toronto (1893–1904) granted the dental degree by examination to successful candidates who had graduated from recognized dental schools. No actual teaching occurred.

K   A summary of recommendations contained in a brief to the Royal
    Commission on Health Services submitted by the Canadian Dental
    Association, March 1962

1 That the Provincial legislatures make mandatory the fluoridation of com-
  munal waters
2 That dental public health educational programs be organized and actively
  promoted in all health regions or units
3 That the amount of money available for dental research be increased
  commensurate with the increased demands of research projects
4 That the provinces institute dental treatment benefits for all beneficiaries
  of presently operating public assistance programs
5 That the Royal Commission on Health Services, in co-operation with the
  dental profession, undertake a definitive study of dental health needs and
  factors influencing demand for dental care
6 That the federal government establish machinery to maintain, through
  annual compilation of dental health data, the dental health index initiated
  by the Canadian Dental Association
7 That immediate planning be undertaken to provide additional dental
  schools at the University of British Columbia, at the University of Saskatchewan, at Laval University, and one additional school in Ontario; that the
  Faculty of Dentistry at Dalhousie University be expanded; and that facilities for training dental hygienists be made available at the University of
  Montreal, McGill University, the University of Manitoba, and at the four
  additional dental schools recommended
8 That federal grants to universities be increased in order to permit dental
  faculties to improve the ratio of full-time staff to part-time staff
9 That health agencies employing dentists adopt dental salary schedules
  comparable to incomes available in private practice
10 That more government funds be made available to universities to enable
  dental schools to expand graduate programs for training specialists and to
  add these programs where they do not now exist
11 That this royal commission undertake a detailed thorough study of recruitment to the health professions
12 That the federal government increase its annual per capita grants to universities sufficiently to permit gradual reduction of fees, beginning with the
  more expensive courses such as dentistry, until, at the earliest opportunity,
  they may be removed entirely

13 That a revolving loan fund be established for undergraduate and post-graduate dental students, with initial capital to be provided by matching contributions of $50,000 each from the Canadian Dental Association and the federal government

14 That federal and provincial income tax regulations be amended to permit tax relief for dentists who attend training courses under auspices of universities or recognized dental associations

15 That dental schools give preference to applicants from rural areas, all other factors being equal, as long as the uneven rural-urban distribution of dentists continues

16 That financial and other inducements be provided to encourage more dentists to settle in municipalities without resident dentists

17 That provincial governments engage full-time travelling dentists to serve areas with populations too scattered to warrant resident dentists

18 That dental schools be provided with the financial support required to carry out pilot studies and operational research to determine the best methods of employing auxiliary personnel

19 That the training of future dental assistants and dental technicians be carried out using clinical facilities of university dental schools

20 That dental departments be established in all public hospitals where dental personnel are available to provide both in-patient and out-patient services

21 That provincial public hospital acts or regulations be amended to permit dentists appointed to hospital staffs to admit patients to hospitals

22 That out-patient dental clinics be established in public general hospitals, especially to assist in meeting the needs of marginal income groups

23 That centres for treatment of cleft palate cases be established in children's hospitals, and in general hospitals where adequate paediatric and associated services are available.

Index

Flanagan, J.C., 211
Flavelle, Sir Joseph, 91
Fluoridation, 242
Focal infection, 170
Foot engine, 63
Forceps, 30
Fortier, Armand, 209, 218

Garvin, Matthew H.: British reciprocity, 184; editor, 193; biographical, 244
Gaudreau, Stanislas, 89, 183
Gidney, Eleazer, 15
Giffard, Robert, 9
Gilbert, Benson, 50
Gies, William J., 165
Giles, William J., 101
Globensky, Stephen, 10, 87
Godsoe, F.A., 104, 116, 195
Gold foil, 30, 51, 63, 134
Gold inlay, 92
Golden Jubilee celebration, 243
Good Samaritan Dental Association, 110
Goodwin, A.H., 68
Goodwin, W.S., 68, 232
Graduate degrees, 183
Graduate education, 223
Grady, L. King, 5
Green, William, 12
Greene, William J., 189
Grieve, George, 226
Grieve Memorial Lecture, 226
Gunsmiths, 19, 36

Hackett, W.T., 151
Halifax, 12
Halifax explosion, 163
Halifax Medical College, 113
Halifax Visiting Dispensary: formation, 32; closure, 175
Hamel, Philippe, 193
Hamilton Dental Society, 53
Hamilton, Ira, 202
Hamilton, W. Scott, 234
Hand instruments, 29
Haggin, Joseph B., 32
Hanna, G.E., 76, 82
Hannah, George O., 117
Harris, Chapin A., 11
Harris, S.M., 32
Hart, E.R.K., 258
Harvard University, 105
Hayden, Horace B., 166

Hayhurst, T.E., 214
Health insurance, 207-11, 226
Health and Welfare, 220
Hébert, Louis, 9
Hemingway, Ernest, 159
Henderson, Thomas, 223
Henry, Frederick G., 142
High speed equipment, 243
Hill, Annie Grant, 88
Hipkins, H., 62
Honey, S.L., 228
Hospitals: dental, 56; mental, 88; payment plans, 250
Hubbard, C.H., 32
Hughes, Sir Sam, 153
Hume, Mr, 12
Hunter, John, 12, 109
Hunter, William, 124
Husband, R.J., 98
Hutton, William L., 242
Hydrogen peroxide, 89
Hygienist, dental: first, 172; legislation, 241; training facilities, 252
Hypnosis, 89

Ibbottson, J.S., 93
Implantation of teeth, 89
Incorruptible Enamel Teeth, 18, 29
Indentureship: Beers contract, 25; abuses, 57, 86; control, 108; demise, 142
Indians, 1-6
Industrial dentistry, 172
Institute Dentaire Franco-American, 110
Instruments, hand, 29
Instruments, manufactured, 30
International Dental Federation, 232
Inventions, 260
Itinerant dentists, 15, 24
Ivory, J.W., 79

Janes, L.V., 220
Johnson, C.N., 76, 192
Jones, E.C., 212
Jones, Thomas J.: career, 70; organizer, 97
Jones, William Allen, 54
Journal of Canadian Dental Association, 193
Journal of the Times, 48
Jury service, 56
Juvet, C.H., 108

Index

Toronto General Hospital, 94, 137
Toronto Painless Dental Parlours, 110
Toronto Trades and Labour Council, 96
Toronto, University of: Royal College
of Dental Surgeons affiliated, 74;
Beers' library, 101, refused to estab-
lish faculty, 137; faculty established,
168; graduate degrees, 183; training of
technicians, 214; specialist training,
224; dental public health course, 228;
research, 230; new enlarged building,
251
Training facilities, 222
Trelford, W.G., 202
Trench mouth, 155
Trestler, C.F.F., 78
Trinity College, University of, 82
Turnkey, 30

United States: dentists from, 12
Upper Canada, 10, 12

Van Buskirk, George, 29
Van Buskirk, Lawrence E., 27–9
Vars (of Oshawa), 84
Veterans Affairs, Department of, 219

Walker, Thomas, 32
Walsh, Arthur L.: appointed dean, 196;
health insurance, 209; portrait, 218;
retired as dean, 234; school survey,
240
Wansbrough, E.M., 221
War Memorial Fund, 222
War Regulations, 214
Watts, John, 12
Webster, Albert E.: editor, 101; sepsis,
123; biological concept, 135; dental
nurse, 160; alteration in dental train-
ing, 167; honorary degree, 192; career
summary, 194
Webster, J.H., 28, 78
Welfare services, 229
Wells, Horace, 29, 53
Wells, John, 88

Wells, S. C. Josephine, 87
West China Mission, 127
Western Canada Dental Society, 108
Western Dental Society, 53
Western Ontario, University of, 251
Wetmore, H.C., 98
White, Samuel S., 31
Williams, C.H.M., 7, 230
Willmott, J.B.: biographical, 58–61;
university affiliation, 74; on profes-
sional maturity, 78; appointed in
charge of school, 81; implantation,
90; comment on local anaesthesia, 93;
planning of school building, 94; need
for national organization, 107; not a
specialty of medicine, 109; death, 140
Willmott, W.E.: early activity, 61; drugs
in use, 89; career summary, 141;
honoured, 195
Wilson, D.D., 219
Wilson, William, 67
Winnipeg, 64
Women dentists: first graduate, 87;
refugees, 215; small percentage, 257
Wood, Henry T.: early dentist, 22;
founder, 40; itinerants, 50; recognition
for superior ability, 63; building of
school, 94
Wood, Samuel, 17
Woodbury, Frank: recognized leader,
99; reciprocity of licence, 104;
Dominion Dental Council, 108;
comment on relationship of dentistry,
109; dean, 113–16; enlarged responsibility for profession, 167
Woodbury, W.W.: family, 113; leadership, 217; orthodontics, 226; retirement as dean, 234
Woods, James, 50
World Health Organization, 232

X-ray, 91, 204

York (Toronto): itinerants, 12; first
resident dentist, 17
Yukon, 110